A Brief
History of
Chinese
Medicine

2nd Edition

A Brief
History of
Chinese
Medicine

2nd Edition

PY Ho

The Needham Research Institute, Cambridge, UK

F P Lisowski

University of Tasmania, Hobart, Australia

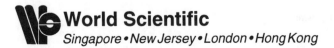
World Scientific
Singapore • New Jersey • London • Hong Kong

Published by

World Scientific Publishing Co. Pte. Ltd.

P O Box 128, Farrer Road, Singapore 912805

USA office: Suite 1B, 1060 Main Street, River Edge, NJ 07661

UK office: 57 Shelton Street, Covent Garden, London WC2H 9HE

British Library Cataloguing-in-Publication Data
A catalogue record for this book is available from the British Library.

A BRIEF HISTORY OF CHINESE MEDICINE, 2nd Edition

ISBN   981-02-2717-5
ISBN   981-02-2803-1 (pbk)

Printed in Singapore.

This account is dedicated to
Dr Philip Mao Wen-Chee
and
Members of the Board
of the
East Asian History of Science Foundation,
Hong Kong
who have done so much in their munificent
support of the Needham Research Institute, Cambridge,
and thereby to the spread of knowledge of the history
of medicine, science and technology of China.

Preface to the Second Edition

In this edition we have changed the title of our little book. In the previous edition we called it *Concepts of Chinese Science and Traditional Healing Arts: A Historical Review*. However, this caused a little confusion in the mind of our readers and therefore we decided that a more appropriate title would be *A Brief History of Chinese Medicine* which expresses more clearly the purpose of our account.

This new edition is a slightly expanded version of the previous one. We added a number of details and brought the recent statistics up to date. The Chinese names have been removed from the text and placed in a separate glossary at the end. A pronunciation guide has also been added. We hope that this brief account of the history of Chinese medicine will be of continued interest and will stimulate readers to look further into the fascinating history of an ancient and evolving culture that has had such major influence in the East Asian region and beyond.

We thank Mrs Sharon Monk of the Department of Anatomy and Physiology for her patience and kindness in word processing this edition which is much appreciated.

We owe warm thanks to our wives Lucy and Ai-yue for their support, encouragement and interest throughout this enterprise.

Again our sincere thanks to Professor K.K. Phua, the Editor-in-Chief, Ms Lim Sook-Cheng, Assistant Director of Publishing, and the staff of World

Scientific Publishing Company in Singapore for their kind interest, support and guidance.

HPY
FPL
Cambridge and Hobart 1996

Preface to the First Edition

The object of this brief introductory discourse is to render homage to some of our far distant predecessors in the craft of medicine in classical Chinese culture. Too often people have taken an unduly narrow view of the history of medicine, confining it to the discoveries of the Greeks and the more ancient nations from whom they learnt, but we must be more oecumenical and celebrate the achievements of their contemporaries in eastern Asia (Needham). Though Chinese civilisation is not so old as those of Babylonia and ancient Egypt, it is much older than that of Greece and Rome, and already it is becoming apparent that some 2 millennia BC the foundations for Chinese medicine were laid.

The main body of this little work deals with the historical development of medicine in China whose influence on Korea, Japan and Southeast Asia was profound and even reached far west into the Islamic world.

The present account had its origins in the University of Hong Kong in the mid-1970s when one of us (FPL) became aware that the medical students whom he was teaching were unacquainted with the rich history of Chinese medicine and only had a perfunctionary notion of the underlying concepts. Several students asked for more information and thus it was decided to prepare some lecture notes on the history of medicine in general with particular emphasis on China and Japan. Subsequently the two authors came together and expanded the original notes for distribution among the students. It was these very students who provided the initial impetus to this little venture. We thank them.

More recently these notes have been reviewed, but no attempt has been made to present an exhaustive study. We want now to try to show something of what China contributed to the world growth of the medical sciences, to acquaint readers working in many different subjects, and at many different levels with a glimpse of the concepts and history of Chinese medicine. We hope they find information and profit in it and will feel encouraged to delve deeper.

Finally there are certain friends and colleagues we have to thank. Firstly we would like to take this opportunity to express our grateful thanks to Dr Joseph Needham, C.H., Sc.D., F.R.S., F.B.A., of the Needham Research Institute, Cambridge, U.K., who provided the indirect stimulus and is in so many ways a mentor to us both.

We acknowledge with gratitude Miss Annie Kwan of the Department of Anatomy, University of Hong Kong, who typed the original drafts and Ms Lee Bradburn of the Department of Physiology, University of Tasmania, who kindly word-processed the expanded drafts and final version.

Our thanks are also due to Professor K.K. Phua, the Editor-in-Chief of World Scientific Publishing Co. in Singapore, and his staff for their kind help and guidance.

HPY
FPL
Cambridge and Hobart 1993

CONTENTS

Introduction

The proper study of medicine involves a study of its history. The development of medicine is not only concerned with the skills and science of the subject, but also with its ethics and education. It is appropriate that aspiring doctors beginning their basic training should have at least an outline knowledge of the history of their subject. Growing interest in the history of medicine is apparent from the large number of contemporary publications.

Before embarking on an outline of the concepts and history of Chinese medicine it is necessary to make some preliminary remarks in order to have a better understanding of the development of health care and its various branches.

From the point of view of the chronological and orderly relation of human facts and ideas, history is but a recent affair in relation to the environment in which it moves. Study of the earliest origins of medical thought and its developmental trends goes back to the most distant periods of the history of humanity, when humans first appeared on the world stage, when their physical, psychological, and social individuality were slowly forming, when the characteristics of the population to which they belonged were scarcely apparent in their essential features.

But even in the period which preceded the appearance of humans on the earth, the investigations of palaeopathology have demonstrated that almost synchronously with the first manifestations of life there is indubitable evidence of disease.

From studies of human skeletal remains it is evident that humans already practised some form of early medicine during the late Palaeolithic period (c. 600 000 to 7000 BC). Since science and magic are in their early stages indistinguishable, it is difficult to differentiate between ritual or magical and therapeutic motives underlying the practice of the healing craft.

For example, it is well known that the surgical practice of trepanation, the removal of a disc of bone from the skull, took place some 10,000 years ago, at the end of the Palaeolithic period. This operation was also practised during the Neolithic age (c. 7000 to 1600 BC). The indications for trepanation were severe headaches (letting out evil spirits) and skull injuries. Most of the examples of this surgical procedure come from central and western Europe. The practice has continued until recent times and was quite widespread. Thus in early and later historic times this type of surgery was performed in ancient Peru, north Africa, western Asia and Oceania. Studies of this period reveal how successful Neolithic humans were. The mortality rate for this serious operation at that time was only between 20 and 30 percent, while during the Middle Ages it amounted to nearly 100 percent. Trepanation was therefore abandoned and only resurrected in the 19th century when asepsis was introduced.

Medicine, which is an applied science, has an ancient history. And in order to understand this development we have to realise that there is no such thing as Western medicine, there is only *one* universal medicine and that is scientific medicine, which is the sum and synthesis of all the world's medical experience. To this people of all cultures and nations have and are contributing. There is only *one* unitary science of Nature (and medicine is part of it) which in its study is approached more or less uniformly, and which is built up more or less successfully and continuously, by various groups of humanity from time to time. This means that one can expect to trace an absolute continuity between the first beginnings of medicine in ancient Babylonia, through the advancing natural knowledge of historic China, India, the Islamic world and the classical Western world to modern times.

Of course humans have always lived in an environment essentially constant in its properties, and their knowledge of it must therefore tend towards a constant structure. But all science, including that of medicine, develops out of one state of theoretical understanding into another. There is no steady state, only a continuous flow with ebbs and tides at different times depending on the pressures that either enhance or depress the flow. In the same manner theories arise, prosper, prevail (often even long after they have been disproved), disappear or even reappear.

The history of medicine is not just a history of discoveries and of illustrious names. A study of the universal comparative history of science and medicine teaches us that the really informative contrasts, as Nathan Sivin suggests, are not those between isolated discoveries, but between those whole systems of thought which have served as the matrices of discoveries. In order to understand this we have to take into account certain basic considerations:

1. the world views and scientific philosophy of ancient and modern times;
2. the relationship of traditional and present day ideas;
3. the milieu and socioeconomic environments in which these ideas developed and prospered (or even regressed); and
4. what pressures these ideas were subjected to.

It is only in this way that one can understand and interpret the past history. The evolution of modern science and medicine can only be causally explained in the context of the various possibilities opened and closed by the totality of ideas, values and social attitudes of their time. Joseph Needham uses the image of the history of the sciences of all peoples and cultures as rivers flowing into the ocean of modern science. In the words of the old Chinese saying: "The rivers pay court to the sea".

Until the time of the European renaissance (14th to 16th century AD), the medicine of Asia was the world's most advanced. Indeed, the main branches — Chinese, Indian (Ayurveda), Arabic (Unani) and Persian — gave rise to a large share of the medical learning that formed the foundation of modern European medicine. Chinese medical concepts had a profound influence on its near and far neighbours: Korea, Japan, Southeast Asia and Persia (thereby penetrating also into the Arab World). Reciprocal influences occurred also between China and India.

Guide to Pronunciation

The *pinyin* system for romanising Chinese was introduced in China in the 1950s. It is now the official romanisation system in the People's Republic of China, and has been adopted by the United Nations and other World agencies, it is now the system most commonly used in scholarship and journalism, largely supplanting the older Wade-Giles system. In most cases the *pinyin* system is pronounced as it looks, the important exceptions being the *pinyin* "c" pronounced as "ts", and the "q", which is pronounced as "ch". The following table shows pronunciations with approximate English equivalents:

a	as in *father*	**n**	as in *no*
b	as in *be*	**o**	like *a* in *raw*
c	like *ts* in *its*	**p**	as in *part*
ch	as in *church*	**q**	like *ch* in *cheat*
d	as in *door*	**r**	as in *red* or like *z* in *azure*
e	as in *her*	**s**	as in *sir*
f	as in *fit*	**sh**	as in *short*
g	as in *go*	**t**	as in *ton*
h	as in *her*	**u**	as in *too*, also as in French
i	like *ea* in *eat* or *i* in *sir*		*tu* or German ü
j	as in *jeep*	**w**	as in *want*
k	as in *kite*	**x**	like *sh* in *sheet*
l	as in *late*	**y**	as in *yes*
m	as in *me*	**z**	as in *zone*

zh	like *j* in *jump*
ai	like *ie* in *tie*
ao	like *ow* in *how*
ei	like *ay* in *hay*
ie	like *ie* in *experience*
ou	like *oe* in *toe*

Part 1

CHINESE MEDICINE: AN OVERVIEW OF ITS CONCEPTS AND HISTORY

Part 1

CHINESE MEDICINE:
AN OVERVIEW OF ITS
CONCEPTS AND HISTORY

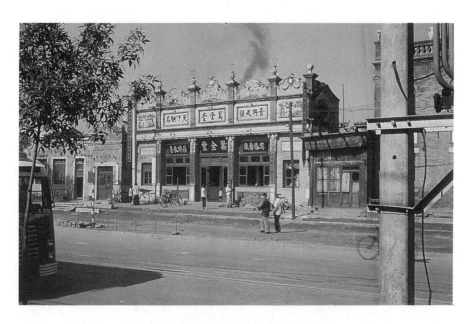

An old pharmacy in Beijing, 1964 (Photo FPL).

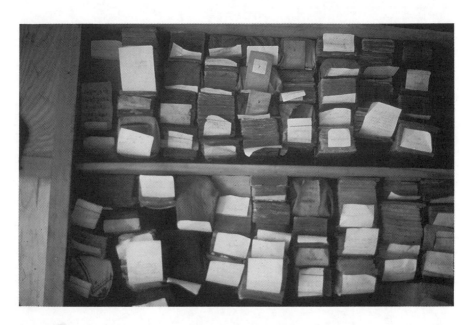

A section of the library, showing Mongolian and Tibetan medical texts at the Mongolian Traditional Medical Research Centre in Xilinhot in 1980 (Photo FPL).

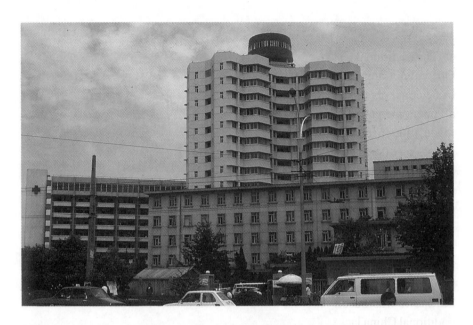

The Traditional Chinese Medical College and Hospital in Chengdu in 1988 (Photo FPL).

The traditional Chinese healing arts form an integral part of Chinese culture. One cannot appreciate Chinese culture fully without taking into account the basic concepts of Chinese thought which were employed to explain not only all phenomena in nature, but also all human activities. Historically China has made immense contributions to medicine in the fields of pharmacology, physiology (such as endocrinology), clinical medicine, public health, medical colleges (including medical education and examination systems), the registration of physicians, acupuncture, moxibustion, and so on. Some of these practices and ideas came to Europe by way of western Asia along the Silk Road and by sea via the Arabs.[1]

For comparative purposes we must realise that for some two thousand years Chinese society was constructed in an entirely different way from anything known in the West. The society was based on bureaucratic feudalism, while in Europe it was based on aristocratic military feudalism. Broadly speaking, traditional China lacked the apparatus of fiefs and feudal ranks, of primogeniture and inherited lordships; instead of all this the Chinese society was governed by a non-hereditary bureaucracy, an immensely elaborate civil service, the members of which were drawn from the ranks of the educated gentry. Instead of earls and barons there were governors and magistrates. Access to this "mandarinate" was by means of official examinations. Thus the *carrière ouverte aux talents* was a Chinese invention which arose a couple of millennia earlier than its successor in France, to quote from Needham. As might be expected, the influence of this very different form of society upon medicine was profound.

The historical foundations of medicine in China are already met with in the 29th century BC and recent work tends to give us even earlier dates. A table of Chinese dynasties is provided (Table 1).

The beginning of Chinese medicine is traditionally attributed to Shennong (The Heavenly Husbandman), the legendary emperor who introduced agriculture and had personally tasted the hundred types of plants in order to discover their medicinal values. He is also supposed to have introduced the technique of acupuncture. For many centuries he has been regarded as the patron sage of Chinese physicians. Shennong is said to have lived about 2700 BC. Nowadays, it is believed that the name Shennong only represented a certain phase in prehistory, when medicine, in its very elementary form, was first used among the early Chinese people. Needles made from animal bones

Table 1   Outline of Chinese Historical Periods

Xia	2200–1700 BC	**Northern**	
Shang	1700–1100* BC	Northern Wei	386–534
Zhou	1100*–221 BC	Eastern Wei	534–550
Western Zho	1100*–771 BC	Western Wei	535–556
Eastern Zhou	770–256 BC	Northern Qi	550–577
Spring & Autumn		Northern Zhou	557–581
Period	770–476 BC		
Warring States		**Sui**	581–618
Period	476–221 BC	**Tang**	618–907
		Five Dynasties	907–960
Qin	221–207 BC	Later Liang	907–923
		Later Tang	923–936
Han	206 BC–220 AD	Later Jin	936–946
Western Han	206 BC–24 AD	Later Han	947–950
Eastern Han	25–220 AD	Later Zhou	951–960
Three Kingdoms Period	220–280	**Liao**	916–125
Wei	220–265	**Song**	960–279
Shu Han	221–263	Northern Song	960–127
Wu	222–280	Southern Song	1127–1279
Jin	265–420	**Western Xia**	1038–1227
Western Jin	265–316	**Jin**	1115–1234
Eastern Jin	317–420	**Yuan (Mongol)**	1271–1368
		Ming	1368–1644
Southern & Northern Dynasties		**Qing (Manchu)**	1644–1911
Southern	420–589		
Song	420–479	**Republic of China**	1912–1949
Qi	579–502	**People's Republic**	
Liang	502–557	**of China**	1949–
Chen	557–589		

*Traditional dates before 841 BC are not firm historical dates. For example, the year for the establishment for the Zhou dynasty has been variously put as 1122 BC, 1100 BC, 1055 BC and 1030 BC.

found at the site of Peking Man in Zhoukoudian suggest their use to sew animal skins together as a cover against the elements, showing that the infancy of preventative medicine had already started about half a million years before our time.[2] From studying the inscriptions on oracle bones, which were tortoise shells and shoulder-blades or scapulae of a species of buffalo, used between the sixteenth and eleventh centuries BC by the Shang people for divination, we know that the Chinese at that time made use of wine and hot water as medicine and bronze knives and needles as surgical instruments. They also knew about intestinal parasites, and believed that tooth decay was caused by worms.

It is believed that in the early stages medicine and magic were indistinguishable and were practised by shamans (*wu*) who are still active among North Asian tribal peoples today. In fact shamans and doctors were referred to together as *"wu yi "* (shamans and doctors). During the Zhou dynasty (11th century BC to 3rd century BC) the post of court physician was already established. During the Spring-and-Autumn Period (722 BC to 480 BC) there were several physicians of great fame, most of whom came from the State of Qin, in modern Shaanxi province. They showed that physicians and shamans had already parted company by that time. We read about He the physician in 540 BC who was sent by the Earl of the State of Qin to attend to the illness of the Marquis of the State of Jin (in modern Shanxi province). His prescription was a lecture given to his patient on moderation as the best remedy for an illness caused by overindulgence in sex.

Then there was the celebrated physician of the Spring-and-Autumn Period, Qin Yueren, better known by the name of Bian Que (fl. 501 BC), who ranked in China as Hippocrates (465 BC to 370 BC) did in Europe, but lived at least one generation earlier than the latter. An account about him is given by Sima Qian in the *Shiji* (Historical Memoirs). We are informed that Bian Que was already acquainted with the four important diagnostic procedures used in Chinese medicine, namely, an observation of external signs shown in the face, eyes, nose, ears, mouth, tongue and throat of the patient *(wang)*; listening to sounds emitted by coughing, breathing and talking, i.e. early forms of auscultation and osphresis (*wen*); taking the patient's history, anamnesis, by inquiring about the site of discomfort, his appetite, his bowels, etc. (*wen*); and finally palpation and pulse-feeling, sphygmology (*qie*). It is said that Bian

Que once visited the palace in the State of Guo (in modern Henan province) and found the Crown Prince unconscious, but pronounced dead by the court physicians. Bian Que went to the Crown Prince, felt his pulse and then asked one of his disciples to assist him to apply acupuncture. Thus he revived the Prince who emerged with the appearance of a person in good health after receiving his treatment. Those who were around were much astonished and spread the words that Bian Que could even cure a person who was already dead. Bian Que in reply said that he did not resurrect a corpse, but only cured a patient. On another occasion Bian Que visited the Marquis of the State of Qi (in modern Shandong province), and from the complexion of the latter he noted that he was looking at a sick man. He told the Marquis his observation, but not having any symptom of discomfort the Marquis did not take heed. Five days later he saw the Marquis again and on looking at his complexion repeated his previous warning and added that his condition had worsened, but again the Marquis would not listen to him. Another five days later he met the Marquis and told him that he could observe that his illness had now become even worse than on the two previous occasions when they saw each other, but again the Marquis maintained that he was in good health and paid no attention to Bian Que. Five days later Bian Que came to see the Marquis and left without uttering a word. Thinking that Bian Que was admitting his own mistake by keeping silent the Marquis sent someone to ask Bian Que why he left without giving any advice to his lordship. Bian Que told the messenger that the illness of the Marquis had reached a stage when no medicine could cure and no amount of acupuncture could have any effect and hence he could not have given any useful advice. Five days later the Marquis fell ill and quickly sent for Bian Que. However, Bian Que had already left; the Marquis died shortly afterwards.

The earliest Chinese medical writing known to us is the *Huangdi neijing suwen* (The Yellow Emperor's Manual of Corporeal Medicine). As its title implies its authorship has been attributed to the legendary Yellow Emperor, Huang Di who has been given the traditional dates of between 2698 and 2599 BC. The book actually consists of two treatises, namely, the *Suwen* (Questions and Answers about Living Matter) and the *Lingshu* (The Vital Axis). The *Suwen* appears to have been written by several unknown authors during the Spring-and-Autumn Period and the Warring States Period (480 BC to 221 BC), and its final form only eventuated during the second century BC in early Western Han.[3] The *Lingshu*, which deals with medical physiology, anatomy and acupuncture, was written during the second century BC and again we are ignorant of its exact authorship or authorships. Between the winter of 1973 and the spring of 1974 some valuable medical writings were discovered during the excavations at Mawangdui near the city of Changsha in modern Hunan province. The tomb where these writings were found dates back to the year 168 BC and hence the medical writings concerned must have belonged to an earlier date. These are the most ancient Chinese medical writings extant.

The traditional Chinese believed in the harmony of nature — the close relationship between heaven (*tian*), earth (*di*), and man (*ren*), the so-called "three forces" (*sancai*). Their world-view conceived a harmonious co-operation of all matters in the universe, arising from the fact that they were all parts of a hierarchy of wholes forming a cosmic and organic pattern and obeying the internal dictates of their own nature. The famous Song neo-Confucianist Zhu Xi (1130 to 1200) identified two fundamental entities of nature, namely, *li* and *qi*, saying, "Throughout the universe there is no *qi* without *li*, nor *li* without *qi* ". Elucidating these two entities he said, "Throughout heaven and earth there is *li* and there is q*i*. *Li* is the *Dao* (that organises) all forms (*xing*) from above and the roots from which all things are produced. *Qi* is the instrument (qi) composing all forms from below, and the tools and raw material with which all things are made. Thus men and all other things must receive this *li* in their moment of coming into existence, and thus obtain their specific nature (*xing*). They must also receive this *qi* in order to get their form (*xing*)." Hence Zhu Xi visualised *li* as something similar to the cosmic and organic pattern and *qi* as something reminding us of our modern concept of matter-energy if not also the ancient ideas of *pneuma* of the Greeks and *prâna* of the Hindus.

Li and *qi* in operation give rise to another entity *shu*, about which Zhu Xi said, "When there is *li* there is *qi*, and when there is *qi* there is *shu*. That is to say *shu* comes between (them)". The word "*shu*" has a very wide range of meanings. In its modern sense it generally refers to "numbers", "mathematics" and "counting", and less frequently it has the sense of "to reprimand", "to discriminate" or "an art". In our present context, however, it embraces not only "mathematics" and "numerology" but also "calendrical science" and "prognostications from the calendar" (*lishu*) and "fate and destiny" of various aspects from the country as a whole to the individual, known differently as *tianshu* (predestination of heaven), *mingshu* (fate), *dingshu* (predestination), and *yunshu* (destiny-cycle). More generally it refers to the way that the forces of nature operate. The mystic philosopher Zhuangzi remarked about the year 290 BC:

> There is something which one gets from without and responds to from within but cannot express in words. It is the *shu* that exists in it.

Bearing Zhuangzi's advice in mind we shall go no further in making a futile attempt to express *shu* in words or to translate it into another language, such as English.

Unlike in Europe, science and the humanities have never parted company in traditional China, where every conceivable object or phenomenon, from astronomy to astrology, from alchemy to magic, from ethics to politics, and from philosophy to the art of healing, was considered to operate under the same principles of *li*, *qi* and *shu*.

Zhu Xi identified *li* as *taiji* (variously rendered as "Supreme Ultimate" and "Supreme Pole"), which is the ultimate source of all things. Zhou Dunyi (1017 to 1073) said:

> The *taiji* moves and produces the *Yang*. When the movement reaches a   limit it comes to rest. The *taiji* at rest produces the *Yin*. When the state of rest comes to a limit it returns to a state of motion. Motion and rest alternate, each being the source of the other. *Yin* and *Yang* take up their appointed function to establish the "Two Forces (*liangyi*). *Yang* is transformed by combining with *Yin*, producing Water, Fire, Wood, Metal and Earth. Then the five *qi* diffuse harmoniously, and the four seasons take their course.
>
> *Yin* and *Yang* are the two components of the primordial *qi*. *Yin*, the negative principle, represents cloudiness, the moon, earth, night, water, cold, dampness, darkness, what is feminine, what is in the passive, the process of contraction, and so forth; while *Yang*, the positive principle, refers to sunshine, the sun, heaven, day, fire, heat, dryness, brightness, what is masculine, what is active, the process of expansion, and so on (Table 2 and Fig. 1).

The true flowering of Chinese medicine began during the time of the two Han dynasties (206 BC to AD 220). Medical schools were founded in various parts of China. It is demonstrable that examinations of scholarly proficiency were inaugurated by the Han emperor Wendi in 165 BC, while the Imperial Academy (*taixue*) was founded in 124 BC. Although the aim of the academy was mainly literary, philosophical and administrative, instructions were also given on the sciences and other subjects that were regarded to be of importance to the state, such as astronomy, hydraulic engineering and medicine. The Han dynasties also saw the beginning of a rudimentary form of a national medical service. It was divided into two divisions, one to attend to the imperial palace and the other to attend to the provincial and medical administration and to the army.

In a bureaucratic society it was quite natural that in the development of the conception of hospitals, religious and governmental initiatives should, from time to time, contend together. The general picture emerges that the idea of the hospital in China first arose in the Han period before the introduction of Buddhism from India. In the year AD 2 following a severe draught and a locust plague an imperial edict ordered that the sick be accommodated in empty buildings and given treatment. There were other similar instances, but there were no permanent institutions. The first permanent hospital with a dispensary was established in the year 491 by Xiao Ziliang, a Buddhist prince of the Southern Qi dynasty. Then in the year 510 Toba Yu, a prince of Northern Wei dynasty, established a government hospital under the Ministry of Imperial Sacrifices (*taichangbu*). This hospital had a distinctly charitable purpose, being intended primarily for the poor or destitute suffering from disabling diseases. Later in the same century we have an example of semi-private benefactions when Xin Gongyi, one of the generals who had conquered the house of Chen and helped to establish the Sui dynasty, encountered a violent epidemic in the province where he retired to be governor. Whereupon he turned his own residence and offices into a hospital and provided medicine and medical attendants for thousands of people. During the 7th century we begin to witness conflict between religious and government control of hospitals. In AD 653 Buddhist monks and nuns and Taoist priests were forbidden to practise medicine. In AD 717 the minister Song Jing memorialised the Tang emperor saying that ever since Changan (modern Xi'an) had been the national capital hospitals there were supposed to be under government control, but because of neglect on the part of government officials the functions of the hospital were taken over more and more by the Buddhists. And by the year 734 government supported orphanages and infirmaries were established in the capital.

Besides the examination system and the hospitals, the bureaucratic society in China also brought about two other interesting institutions. One of them was the introduction of quarantine regulations. In the year AD 356 a disastrous epidemic resulted in the emperor of the Jin dynasty applying what were called the "old rules", prohibiting officials whose families had three or more cases from attending court for 100 days. During the 6th century the Indian monk Narendrayasas established leprosaria at the capital of the Sui dynasty for men and women for the isolation of lepers.

We must now return to the Han dynasties. The earliest Chinese pharmacopoeia extant appeared during this period. This is the *Shennong bencaojing* (Pharmacopoeia of the Heavenly Husbandman) which was compiled in the 1st and 2nd century BC during the Western Han period. It is attributed to the legendary emperor Shennong, although no one knows who exactly wrote it. This pharmacopoeia explains the *Yin* and *Yang* and the indications of each medicinal substance and notes that certain combinations of two or more different substances will have a beneficial effect while other combinations will be counter-indicative. The book includes 365 items of medicine of mineral, plant and animal origin, dividing them into three categories. Those in the first are believed to have the efficacy of nourishing or prolonging life; those in the second are generally non-toxic and are used to restore the constitution of the patient; and those in the third category are mostly toxic or have side-effects, and are used for combating diseases.[6] One has to note that the physicians in China were never affected by the Galenic orthodoxy which permitted the use of only plant drugs and they never recognised the association between toxicity and beneficial action. The use of medicine of mineral origin, to be administered orally, such as antimony and mercury, was a subject of great debate during the time of Paracelsus in 16th century Europe. The Chinese pharmacopoeias, from the very beginning as we know them, contain medicinal substances of plant, mineral and even animal origin, while medical prescriptions show that the Chinese physicians had no inhibition in prescribing medicine of mineral origin.

They were aware of the toxicity of some of the substances they used and they seemed to appreciate the intimate association between high toxicity and powerful beneficial action which was to impress Paracelsus so greatly many centuries afterwards.

Western historians attribute the first true *materia medica* text to Dioscordides and Galen in the first and second centuries AD, respectively, but Chinese texts of comparable value (and with many similarities) predated those Greek and Roman healers by many centuries.

In the history of military health care, the Chinese contribution is at least as important as anything which one can find in ancient Greece and Rome. For instance, we now have in the bamboo tablets of army administration, which have been preserved in the sands of the Gobi Desert along the Great Wall, at least as much information about the military medical service of the Han armies as we have about those attached to the legions of Rome. We even have details of their standard prescriptions dating from the 3rd century AD.

There were a number of eminent physicians flourishing during the period of the Han dynasties. Chunyu Yi (205 BC to ?) made careful records of medical case histories. We can read about him from his biography in Sima Qian's *Historical Memoirs*, where his other name, Canggong, is used instead. During that period new influences began to show themselves in Chinese medicine. These were the intrusions of scholars, some of whom also included the study of medicine within their province of learning. Confucianism had something to do with this. The teaching of filial piety encouraged many scholars to study the medical writings so that they might be able to attend to their own parents in time of illness should a physician be unavailable. One effect of the intrusion was the elevation of the literary standard of medical writing and the social status of medical practitioners, but another effect was the introduction of philosophical speculations into medicine to take the place of practical experiments and observations.

In the latter half of the second century of our era Zhang Ji (AD 150 to 219), better known as Zhang Zhongjing, wrote the *Shanghan zabinglun* (Discourse on Fevers and Miscellaneous Illnesses), which since the time of the Song dynasty (960 to 1279) has been separated into two different books, namely one on fevers under the title *Shanghanlun* (Treatise on Febrile Diseases), and the other on dietetics and other sicknesses under the title *Jinkui yaolue* (Essential

Treasury of Medicine). The life and work of Zhang Ji is closely paralleled to that of Galen (AD 131 to 201), for his *Shanghalun* had a profound influence on Chinese medicine and is considered to be the most important medical classic after the *Huangdi neijing suwen*.

In the early third century lived the famous physician and surgeon Hua Tuo (c. 190 to 265), a younger contemporary of Zhang Ji. Hua Tuo is featured in the well-known novel *Sanguo yanyi* (Romance of the Three Kingdoms) as having performed an operation on the right arm of the Shu Han general Guan Yu and was later imprisoned by Cao Cao after he suggested that the latter should undergo neurosurgery for treatment of a severe and persistent pain in the head. He was said to have produced general anaesthesia by the use of wine called *mafeisan*, of which we do not know the exact composition. Indian hemp has been suggested by Miyashita Saburô, but this can only be speculation.[7] Hua Tuo was noted not only for his skill in surgery but also for his development of physiotherapy and medical gymnastics. He became regarded as a patron sage of medicine. He is one of the three deities worshipped at the Sanshenggong Joss-house at Breakfast Creek in Brisbane, Australia.

Considerable development in Chinese medicine took place between the 3rd and 10th century. First, Huangfu Mi (215 to 282) wrote the *Zhenjiu jiayijing* (Systematic Manual of Acupuncture), a major work on acupuncture — a system most characteristic of therapy in Chinese medicine. As we have already noted, Bian Que himself used this method to cure the unconscious prince during the Spring-and-Autumn Period and acupuncture is described earlier in the *Huangdi neijing suwen*. Modern archaeological studies have found specimens of acupuncture needles in a Han tomb. Traditional Chinese medicine identifies a large number of points, varying from over three hundred to over six hundred, on the surface of the human body into some of which the acupuncturist inserts needles of various length and thickness and in various ways as a method of therapy. These points (*xue*) are connected by "tracts", some of which are called *jing* (cardinal tracts) and others called *luo* (decuman tracts). Needham suggests that the Chinese system of acupuncture could have originated out of the phenomenon of referred pain. The ancient Chinese physicians were probably singularly impressed by the relations of transitory pain in the extremities or trunk with passing malfunctions of the viscera. One suggestion to explain the physiological and biochemical effect of acupuncture is that the needles may stimulate the production of antibodies by the reticuloendothelial system, possibly by indirect stimulation through the autonomic nervous system. There may be a neurosecretory effect mediated through the autonomic nervous system upon the suprarenal cortex inducing a rise in cortisone production or a neurosecretory influence upon the pituitary gland. We also know that acupuncture influences the production of endorphins.

Traditional Chinese medicine, however, talks about acupuncture in terms of the *Yin* and *Yang* theory. It identifies twelve cardinal tracts running along the length of the limbs, with six of these tracts categorised as *Yin* and the other six as *Yang*. These twelve tracts pertain to the viscera of the body. There are eight extra cardinal tracts (*mai*) along the head and the trunk interlacing with the twelve cardinal tracts (*jing*) and regulating the *qi* and blood in the latter. The *renmai* is the confluence of all the *Yin* tracts, while the *dumai* is that for all the *Yang* tracts. There are decuman tracts to communicate between the *Yin* and the *Yang* cardinal tracts. The connecting points of the decuman tracts and the cardinal tracts are used in treating diseases which involve both the *Yin* and the *Yang* related cardinal tracts.

In China indisputable textual evidence exists to prove that the circulation of the blood was an established doctrine by the 2nd century BC at the latest. It was conceived that two separate circulations of fluids existed in the body: blood pumped by the heart flowed through arteries, capillaries and veins; and *qi*, a rarefied form of energy which was pumped by the lungs to circulate through the body in invisible tracts. The ancient Chinese recognised that the different types of pulse emanated from the pumping heart. The Dutch East India physician, Wilhelm ten Rhyne, stated in his book of 1685, *Mantissa Schematica de Acupunctura*, that the circulation of the blood was one of the basic tenets of the whole of Chinese medicine.

Pulse-reading has always been an important technique employed by the traditional Chinese physician for the purpose of diagnosis. The first book on this subject was written in the 3rd century by Wang Shuhe (265 to 317). This was the famous medical canon, the *Maijing* (Manual on the Pulses). The technique of pulse-reading developed gradually since the time of Wang Shuhe. Generally speaking, in pulse-reading or rather pulse-feeling, the tips of the index finger, the middle finger and the ring finger of the right hand of the physician are placed lightly over the radial artery at the wrist of the patient. The three positions, the first beginning from the wrist joint and each separated by a finger's breadth, are known as *cun*, *guan*, and *che* respectively. The behaviour of the pulse in these three positions at both wrists, taking into account its rate, its rhythm, its pressure, its volume, and the variation in the pulse wave, as felt by the three fingers, is used by the physician to tell the nature of the illness. According to the theory of pulse-reading, the six positions in the two wrists felt by the fingers also tell the physician about the behaviour of different parts of the human anatomy. No fewer than 51 types of pulse were distinguished.[8] Besides pulse-reading the Chinese had also other diagnostic techniques, such as the examination of the abdomen (*fuzhen*), examination of the back (*anbei*), and inspection of the tongue (*yanshe*). It was taught that there are 37 different appearances of the tongue.

Even the idea of circadian hythms is not foreign to ancient Chinese thinking. Various cyclical features were well known to the ancient practitioners. Menstrual and ovulating cycles are the most obvious, but there were others, such as the variations in the severity of diseases, body temperatures and sensitivity to pain that varied at different times of the day and night.

It was mentioned earlier that about the Spring-and-Autumn Period the physicians had parted company with the shamans. However, while the physicians occupied themselves treating the sick some of the shamans were pursuing the course of avoiding physical death by various ways and means. Some of them attempted to prolong the human life span indefinitely through the preparation and ingestion of elixirs of life. Those were the alchemists, many of whom were well-versed in medicine. Indeed there are many similarities between medical and elixir prescriptions in their basic principles. One of the greatest alchemists of all time was Ge Hong (261 to 341), who was also a celebrated physician of the early 4th century. To him we owe the *Jinkui yaolue* (Prescriptions in the Treasury of Medicine) and the *Zhouhou jiuzufang* (Handbook of Medicine for Emergencies). Prescriptions for various types of diseases, including infectious diseases, smallpox, eye trouble, ailments of women and children are mentioned in these books. We shall come across other alchemists who were at the same time great physicians in their own right, such as Tao Hongjing and Sun Simiao both of whom we shall presently encounter. Chinese alchemy is based also on exactly the same principles of *Yin* and *Yang* and the five *xing*'s as explained above.

The Chinese were well aware of deficiency diseases centuries before the West. This awareness was based on their view of the existence of a balance in nature and consequently of a balance in the diet. Already in the fourth century BC there were Imperial Dieticians. The ancient practitioners were aware of the disease beriberi and were able to treat it with soya beans and milk. They believed that many diseases could be cured by diet alone.

About the year AD 470, a book on the preparation of medicinal substances, entitled the *Leigong paozhi* (The Venerable Master Lei's Book on the preparation of Medicinal Substances) was written by Lei Xiao (AD 420 to 479).

A little later came the celebrated alchemist and Taoist physician Tao Hongjing (451 to 536), who wrote the pharmacopoeia *Bencaojing jizhu* (Collected Annotations of the Pharmacopoeia). This was the most comprehensive and practical compendium of its time. A 5th-century manuscript copy of this pharmacopoeia is still extant. He also wrote the *Zhouhou baiyifang* (Handbook of Medicine for the Hundred Emergencies). Another book entitled the *Mingyi beilu* (Informal Records of the Famous Physicians) is also attributed to him. Many of the drugs listed in Tao Hongjing's books are still being employed today. Among those used in his time were *ephedra* for asthma, ergot for uterine disturbances, sex hormones from animal organs, *dichroa febrifuga* for malaria, aconite as a heart stimulant, *datura* and *cannabis* (marijuana) for anaesthetics, *scopolia* as a sedative and chaulmoogra oil for leprosy. Others of no less antiquity are senna, castor oil, opium, camphor, wormwood and *nux vomica* (strychnine), as well as most of the medicines of mineral origin found in pharmacies today. Just before entering the Tang dynasty, in the year 610, Chao Yuanfang and his collaborators wrote a vast medical treatise entitled the *Zhubingyuan houlun* (On the Origins and Symptoms of Diseases) dealing with many kinds of diseases, including scabies, certain eye diseases, kidney and bladder calculi, infectious hepatitis, etc.[9]

The Chinese in some ways anticipated modern biochemistry. They were predisposed by their manner of thought and a long tradition to view the body as producing powerful biologically active substances. By the 2nd century BC they were isolating sex and pituitary hormones from human urine and using them for medicinal purposes. At least ten different methods were used in obtaining these hormones between 1025 and 1833. In the process the ancient practitioners commenced with simple evaporation and then turned to the method of sublimation, which was familiar to them from alchemy. They also discovered that steroid hormones are stable below their melting-points. Another technique that was used in extracting hormones was the use of chemicals to precipitate them out of the urine. These hormones were used to treat a wide variety of diseases relating to the sex organs, such as impotence, hypogonadism, spermatorrhea and dysmenorrhea.

By the 7th century AD the Chinese were using thyroid hormone to treat goitre. For this thyroid glands of various animals, including sheep and pigs, were used. The method involved air-drying the glands to reduce them to powder, which was taken every night in wine. Seaweed was also used in the treatment of goitre. The latter knowledge was later transmitted to the West. This use of seaweed is first mentioned in the West by Roger of Sicily in his *Practica Chirurgiae* in 1180.

Diabetes is first mentioned in the 7th century AD by the physician Zhen Quan who died in 643. In his book *Gujin lu yanfang* ("Old and New Tried and Tested Prescriptions"), which apparently was lost, and which was quoted by Wang Tao in 752, Chen describes how diabetic patients suffer intense thirst and excrete large amounts of urine which is sweet to the taste.

Medicine did not develop in China in complete isolation. A'soka (273 to 232 BC) despatched eighteen Buddhist monks to the Chinese capital Xianyang (near modern Xi'an, Shaanxi province). However, the visitors were put in prison on the orders of emperor Qin Shihuangdi, and thus no cultural contact could be expected from those who sank into oblivion under such conditions. It was the Han emperor Lingdi (AD 168 to 189) who first officially welcomed Buddhist monks to his court, more out of a desire to acquire the elusive elixir of life which the Daoists in China had not been able to provide him and therefore the hope that the situation could be rectified by consulting Daoists of a different kind, rather than his interest in the teaching of Buddhism. This did not prevent the introduction of Buddhism to China, and in its wake came Indian medicine. Medicine in ancient India was developed by the Brahmans and during the 4th century BC there had also been contact with Greek culture as a result of the invasion by Alexander the Great. Brahmanical medicine came to China with Buddhist writings which were brought in by the monks who generally equipped themselves with at least some knowledge of medicine for their travel over extended periods of time on foreign soil. For example, the catvâri mahâbhûtâvi, which probably bears some influence of the Greek Four Elements, appeared in Chao Yuanfang's *Zhubingyuan haolun* mentioned earlier and also in Sun Simiao's *Qianjing yaofang* soon to be referred to. The most notable contribution to Chinese medicine was perhaps Brahmanical ophthalmology with which the sacred name Nâgârjuna was associated. A number of writings on the subject bear the name Longshu (Dragon Tree), Longmen (Fierce Dragon), either alone or with the title Bodhisattva. A reminder of the Chinese obsession with the elixir of life is the Brahmanical panacea found in the Chinese literature, the Ajiatuo, named after Tathâgata, one who has attained the goal of enlightenment. Buddhist precepts associated health with one's actions and misdeeds in previous lives. This found ready acceptance by the Chinese in general and even by the Daoists, who also assimilated yoga into their own meditation exercise.

We saw earlier that the Imperial Academy was established in the year 124 BC and that instructions in medicine were given there. In AD 493 chairs and lectureships in medicine were established in the Academy. And in Tang China (618 to 907) we witness that the tradition of a government medical institution was already firmly established. In the year 624, for example, the Imperial Medical College (taiyishu) had an establishment of one professor, one assistant professor, twenty medical officers, one hundred auxiliary staff, two pharmacists and forty students in its clinical medicine department; one professor, one assistant professor, ten medical officers, twenty auxiliary staff, and twenty students in its acupuncture department; one professor, four medical officers, sixteen auxiliary staff, and fifteen students in its physiotherapy department; and so on. Between the years 620 and 630 an Imperial Medical College was established together with the establishment of medical colleges in the chief provincial cities. These medical schools had long and difficult courses with many examinations. From that time onwards they also awarded medical degrees.

Although the Chinese were far ahead of others in the matter of qualifying examinations one has to note that these examinations were not meant in China to turn medical practice into an exclusive profession. There were many other ways of becoming a doctor besides having to go through the Academy. One could become a physician by learning from another physician serving as an apprentice; one could also become a physician by working in a pharmacy and studying the prescriptions made by other doctors; and a physician could even be self-taught. The basic texts that had to be studied were generally the *Huangdi neijing suwen*, the *Shanghanlun* of Zhang Ji, the *Mojing* of Wang Shuhe, and one of the pharmacopoeias, depending on the time (for example it would be the *Shennong bencaojing* say, in the 3rd century AD, but it would become the *Bencao gangmu* in the 16th century). The aspiring physician might have gone a step further by studying another text written by Zhang Ji, namely the *Jinkui yaolue* (Systematic Treasury of Medicine) and the case histories written by famous physicians in the past. Hence anybody was allowed to practice medicine from the physician-royal and the group of government physicians trained in the Imperial Academy to those who called themselves "scholar physicians" *ruyi*, and even to the wandering medical pedlars, who went about ringing their special kind of bell on a staff and handing out herbal remedies for the smallest fees.

From the 8th century onwards there was considerable contact between China and the Arab World. The year AD 931 constitutes a focal point in transmission westwards of the principle of qualification for practice, for that was the date of the first qualifying examinations in the Arab World, decreed by the Caliph al-Muqtadir at Bagdad under the superintendence of the eminent physician Sinān ibn-Thābit ibn-Qurrāh is known of Chinese-Arabic contacts during the preceding two centuries, and there is no difficulty in supposing that the Arabs were taking up energetically a much older Chinese idea. The concept of examinations finally went to the West when in the year 1140 Roger of Sicily passed laws concerning state examinations for physicians, and in the year 1224 the medical school in Salerno began to graduate students as *Doctor Medicinae*. It looks as if the Arabic and Western worlds borrowed the idea of examinations in medicine from the Chinese culture just as civil service examinations in the 19th century so long afterwards were introduced with full knowledge of the age-old Chinese parallel in mind. It would hardly be possible to imagine a deeper effect of the environing culture on medicine than this "bureaucratization" of medical knowledge, which had the extremely happy effect of protecting people at large from the activities of ignorant physicians.

Early in the Tang dynasty an imperial edict was passed for the compilation of an official pharmacopoeia. This is the first time that an official pharmacopoeia was ever compiled under government sponsorship. The *Xinxiu bencao* (The New Pharmacopoeia), completed in the year 659 by a team of twenty headed by Su Jing, is the first extant official *materia medica* in the world. This official patronage given to animals and plants in the Tang dynasty was even surpassed by the interest extended to medical prescriptions. In the year 728 the Tang emperor Xuanzong himself composed the *Guangjifang* (General Formulary of Prescriptions), and in the year 796 another Tang emperor, Dezong, published the *Zhenyuan guanglifang* (Valuable Prescriptions of the Zhenyuan reign-period).

An important feature of the bureaucratic society was the rational systematisation in the writing of the many Chinese pharmacopoeias, which are really pharmaceutical natural histories. The first of these, the *Shennong bencaojing* (Pharmacopoeia of the Heavenly Husbandman) which was referred to earlier, was not produced under imperial auspices. However, many later pharmacopoeias, some of which were considerable in size, were compiled on the order of the emperors. Similar works followed over the next ten centuries. What was true of plants and animals was also true of books of standard prescriptions. By the 7th century the systematisation of plants and animal drugs and prescriptions was extended to diseases. Chao Yuanfang in his treatise systematically classified pathological states according to the ideas of the time, without giving any attention to therapeutic methods. Indeed, traditional China was particularly strong in the classificatory sciences, and the modern term for science in Chinese is "kexue", which was first adopted in the 19th century, and means nothing other than "classification of knowledge".

Traditional Chinese medicine had already made contact with the outside world long before the Tang dynasty. For example, many medicinal plants from West Asia were introduced to China by Zhang Qian in the second century before our era, and doctors were sent from China to Korea and Japan during the 6th century AD.[10] However, the Tang dynasty witnessed much more frequent export of Chinese medicine to Korea, Japan and Vietnam and the mutual interchange of medical knowledge with India and the Arab World. Some specimens of Chinese medicine exported to Japan during the 8th century are still preserved today in the imperial Shôsôin. Many Chinese medical books, including almost all the titles that we have just mentioned, were transmitted to Korea and Japan. Many local herbs from Korea and from Vietnam were brought to China, for example ginseng, *Jatropha janipha*, Lour (*bai fuzi*), Korean pine, and *Corydalis ambigua*, Cham et Sch. (*xuan husuo*) from Korea and Sappan wood, cloves, and vanilla grass from Vietnam. In the year 733 several Japanese monks came to study in China, and ten years later they invited a Chinese monk named Jianzhen (or Ganjin in Japanese) to go to Japan to preach Buddhism and to teach medicine, architecture and other techniques. After six attempts over a period of ten years Jianzhen eventually arrived in Japan with a group of disciples and started teaching at Nara, where he later died in the year 763. Many Chinese herbs, such as *Pachyma cocos*, Fr. (*fuling*), *Angelica polymorpha*, Maxim. var. sinensis (*danggui*), *Polygala tenuifolia*, Willd. (*yuanzhi*), *Euphedra sinica*, Stapf. (*mahuang*), etc. went from China to India, while Indian medical works, especially those on eye diseases, were imported to China. Trade between Tang China and the Arab World brought to China medicinal plants like *Pistacia khinjuk*, Stocks (*ruxiang*), myrrh, dragon's blood, *Rosa banksiae*, R.Br. (*muxiang*) and Fenugreek seed. Many plants and medicines from China were in turn exported to the Arab countries. The great Spanish Muslim botanist Ibn al-Baitar (1197 to 1248) mentions in his *Kitab al-Jam fil-Adviya al-Mufrada* many substances of Chinese origin. Among the medicines going from China to the Arab World were rhubarb and cinnamon, and Islamic remedies also went to China.

It was also during the Tang dynasty that the Nestorians, noted for their medical skill, established themselves near the Chinese capital Changan (modern Xi'an). Chinese literature does not provide much information on the Nestorians. In 1625 an 8th century Nestorian stone tablet bearing inscriptions, partly in Syriac but mainly in the Chinese language, came to light. It mentions the arrival of the Nestorian patriarch Ôlophen in the Chinese capital in the year 635 and his warm reception. He was granted permission by the Tang emperor to reside in a temple in the western suburb, where he and his followers translated Syriac texts into Chinese. Although the stone tablet does not mention medicine directly, it does refer to one of the Nestorians named Yi-Si with the words "the sick were attended to and restored". Texts translated by the Nestorians found in the Dunhuang manuscripts mentioned the Greek Four Element theory, medical treatment similar to that practised in ancient Greece and Rome, and Christian teachings concerning the sick. The *Xinxiu bencao* pharmacopoeia includes an ancient Roman medicine called theriaca, which was probably brought to China by the Nestorians.

Many advances in medicine in the direction of clinical medicine, gynaecology, paediatrics, surgery and physiotherapy were also made in Tang China. In dentistry amalgam was used as a filling for tooth cavities. The most famous medical writer of early Tang was perhaps Sun Simiao (581? to 682), who, as we have noted earlier, was also a great alchemist.[11] We do not know his exact date of birth. Some say that he lived to the age of 180 and some said that he lived just over a hundred years. Known popularly as Yaowang (King of Medicine), there are temples dedicated to him in China. He wrote two vast medical treatises, one entitled *Qianjinfang* (The Thousand Golden Remedies) and the other *Qianjin yifang* (Supplement to the Thousand Golden Remedies). He is also remembered for his advice on medical ethics.

In the Han period Zhang Ji wrote in his *Shanghanlun* that in medicine one should first cure one's own superiors and relatives, secondly help the poor and humble, and lastly one should look after one's own health. Confucian influence was very strong in Chinese medical ethics. Sun Simiao must have been under such influence when he wrote:

> I searched the reason why medicine was introduced by the wise
> sages and found that the purpose was to teach every family and
> inform every individual that it would not be loyal nor filial if one
> was unable to cure the illness of the emperor or one's own parent.

Sun Simiao then went on to say that when a physician attended to his patient he should compose himself, ban all his desires and approach the case dedicated to the relief of the sufferings with a compassionate heart. No regard should be given to the social status of the patient, be it lowly or exalted, poverty-stricken or affluent, aged or young, ugly or beautiful, or to his being a friend or enemy, a relative, a Chinese or a foreigner, a wise person or a fool; but everyone should be treated alike, exactly like a close and dear relative. A physician should not consider his own safety, but must regard the sufferings of the patient as his own, so that he was similarly grieved. He must not entertain any desire of just putting on a show, but must be single-minded in his intentions to relieve sufferings. Thus he should not avoid difficulties in travelling, nor should he be concerned with the time, be it day or night, winter or summer. Neither should he be concerned with his personal comfort, whether hungry or thirsty, tired or exhausted. In this way he would truly become a great physician for his people.

The above is only part of what Sun Simiao had to say about the code of a physician, but that will be sufficient for us to draw comparison with the Hippocratic Oath. The great difference between Western and Chinese medical ethics is that the former is being enforced by professional bodies, such as a medical council and a medical association, whereas in the case of the latter there has not been any legal enforcement with power vested in any particular organisation to penalise the individual practitioner other than the criminal court itself. The ethical code of the Chinese physician is therefore a moral issue, observed individually and dependent on one's own conscience, and no uniformity or level can be found in any group.

Chinese medicine has always been governed by the teaching of Confucius since the time of the great sage. Confucian teaching, in brief, is concerned with five moral principles *ren, yi, li, zhi* and *xin*, which, as we can observe, are very strongly reflected in the medical codes propounded by Sun Simiao. *Ren* is the perfect virtue and the ideal of Confucius. It is the inner love of human kind that prompts us to just action without any selfish motive, and it embraces the meanings conveyed by the words love, charity, benevolence and humanity. In fact one Chinese definition of medicine says, "medicine is the art of *ren*" — as the often used saying *yi zhe renshu* goes. The word *yi* symbolises offering oneself like a lamb in a sacrificial ceremony and conveys the meaning of sacrificing oneself in duty to one's neighbour, and embraces the meaning of righteousness, public spirit, loyalty to one's superior and country. *Li*, originally meaning religious liturgy and ceremony, refers here to propriety and proper conduct. *Zhi* is wisdom and knowledge, and acknowledged attribute to the modern medical practitioner that requires no further elaboration. *Xin* conveys the meanings of sincerity, reliability, honesty and trustworthiness, another attribute expected of our modern doctors. Originally Confucianism was never meant to be a kind of religion. *Ren* the innate love for human kind was its only motive force, which was later reinforced by the neo-Confucian interpretation that such a force was also inherent in nature itself. Reward and punishment were not alluded to. Hence Buddhist teaching relating sicknesses with human action, referred to earlier, found ready acceptance in China. It was modified and adopted by the Daoists, until eventually it became assimilated into Chinese culture itself.

One of Sun Simiao's disciples, Meng Shen (621 to 714), was also a noted alchemist and physician. He was the author of the *Shiliao bencao* (Nutritional Therapy; a Pharmacopoeia of Natural History). Other medical writings of special significance include Chen Cangqi's *Bencao shiyi* (Supplement to the Pharmacopoeia) written between AD 731 and AD 741 and Wang Tao's *Waitai miyao* (Important Medical Prescriptions Revealed by the Governor of a Distant Province), written in the year 752. Wang Tao also had an interest in veterinary science. Wang Bing, a contemporary of Wang Tao, wrote commentaries on many of the Chinese medical classics, including the *Maijing* on the pulses.

Chinese medicine made further advances during the Song dynasty (960 to 1279). When Confucianism regained its strength towards the end of the Tang, and especially during the Song dynasty, the national medical service took over more and more of the various hospitals. Within the Imperial Medical College a bureau of public health was set up, called the *Hanlin yiguanyuan*, which at one time comprised a staff of over one thousand. The number of students at that college was set at three hundred.

The first important work of the Song period was the official pharmacopoeia produced by a team of scholars led by Ma Zhi in the year 973. Entitled the *Kaibao bencao* (Kaibao Reign-Period Pharmacopoeia), it was revised in the following year. In the year 1057 it was again revised and enlarged, and was issued under the abbreviated title *Jiayou bencao* (Jiayou Reign-Period Pharmacopoeia). Then in the year 1061 Su Song and his collaborators produced a new official pharmacopoeia called the *Bencao tujing* (Illustrated Pharmacopoeia). There were also several pharmacopoeias that were not written under government sponsorship. The most notable of these pharmacopoeias was the *Zhenglei bencao* (Classified Pharmaceutical Natural History), compiled by Tang Shenwei around the year 1082. It became so successful that it was accepted and turned into an official pharmacopoeia after being given a new title *Daguan bencao* (Daguan Reign-Period Pharmacopoeia). It was subsequently revised, first in 1116, then in 1159, and finally in 1249, each time assuming a new title. Another important pharmacopoeia of that period is the *Bencao yanyi* (Dilations Upon Pharmaceutical Natural History), produced by Kou Zongshi in the year 1116.

The early Chinese medical classics were further developed during the Song period. For example Liu Wansu (1110 to 1200) wrote commentaries on the *Huangdi neijing suwen* and the *Shanghanlun*. Zhang Congzheng (1156 to 1228), better known under his literary name Zhang Zihe, initiated a new method of therapy by putting emphasis on the inducement of perspiration, emesis and purging, especially on the last.

Advances in the study of human anatomy came with the further development of acupuncture. In the year 1026 Wang Weiyi was ordered by the Song emperor Renzong to construct a life-size figure, the interior of which was fitted with models of the organs and viscera, surrounded with water, and the exterior of which was filled with holes to represent acupuncture points set out according to the description given by Sun Simiao. A facsimile of this figure is preserved in Beijing. To describe his model Wang Weiyi wrote the *Tongren tuxuezhenjiu tujing* (Diagrammatic Illustrations of the Acupuncture Points on the Bronze Figure). In later years several other books on acupuncture also made their appearance.

Forensic medicine, too, made considerable progress. An important work on this subject under the title *Xiyuanlu* (Washing Away of Wrongs) written by Song Ci appeared in the year 1247. This is one of the earliest books in the world on forensic medicine, and has already been translated into at least five different European languages.[12]

Attention was paid to occupational diseases, for example, mercury and lead poisoning. There were also further developments in Song China in the preparation of male steroid hormones from urine. The term *ganmao* was also used for the first time in China for influenza and the common cold. Medicine became so popular during the Song dynasty that even many high-officials and scholars became quite proficient in medicine. Among them may be mentioned the astronomer, mathematician and naturalist Shen Gua (1031 to 1095) and the great poet Su Shi (1036 to 1101), who is better known by his literary name

Su Dongpo. Both of them have left behind some notable medical writings, and incidentally it may be mentioned that Su Dongpo himself was also knowledgeable in alchemy although we have no evidence that he ever attempted to make gold or to ingest an elixir of life.

There were a number of famous physicians who lived during the last years of the Song period and the early days when China was conquered by the Mongols. Li Gao (1180 to 1251), also known from his style as the Elder of Dongyuan, or Li Dongyuan, theorised that the stomach and the spleen were the two most important organs to attend to in therapy. The stomach corresponded to *Yang* and the spleen to *Yin*. One must protect the former against *Yin* and the latter against *Yang*. Another great physician was Wang Haogu (fl. 1231 to 1325), whose medical expertise earned him great fame.

During the Song period there was a marked increase in transmission of medical knowledge with India and the Arab World. With the rise of the Mongols in the 13th century, intercultural exchange was further enhanced. In the year 1292 a Muslim pharmacy was set up in the capital Beijing. At about the same time a Chinese translation of some Arabic medical texts, called the *Huihui yaofang* (Muslim Prescriptions) also appeared. From China the art of acupuncture and certain commodities, such as ginger, tea, rhubarb and cinnamon, which are also used in Chinese medicine, were brought to the Arab World. At the same time the Mongols conquered Persia and Iraq, and as a result medical organisations of Arabic type and tradition were added to that of China. The Yuan (Mongol) dynasty (1260 to 1368) produced many books on *materia medica*, paediatrics, nutrition and medical history. Among them we ought to mention the book on acupuncture by Hua Shou, also known under his literary name Boren, namely the *Shisijing huahui* (Elucidations of the Fourteen Acupuncture Tracts), written in the year 1341. This book found its way to Japan and remained apparently lost to the Chinese until a few centuries later when it returned to China with a Japanese commentary. Actually Hua Shou lived in the latter half of the Yuan period and the early part of the Ming dynasty (1368 to 1644), and there were also several famous physicians who lived during this period. Wang Lu, also known by his literary name Wang Andao, had written a number of books commenting on the *Shanghanlun*. Ni Weide (1303 to 1377) introduced many new prescriptions and later became the physician-royal in the service of the first Ming emperor.

Medical writings continued to flourish during the Ming dynasty (1368 to 1644). One of the princes, Zhu Su (1361 to 1425), the fifth son of the first Ming emperor, wrote the *Jiuhuang bencao* (Famine Relief Pharmacopoeia) in 1406.[13] Zhu Su also compiled the *Puzhifang* (Prescriptions for the Multitudes), which contains 61,739 medical prescriptions. One of Zhu Su's sons, Zhu Youdun (1379 to 1439) compiled a vast compendium of medical prescriptions known as the *Xiuzhenfang* (Handy Prescriptions). A book on alchemy entitled the *Gengxin yuce* (Precious Secrets about Metals and Minerals) written by another prince, Zhu Quan (1377 to 1448) is frequently quoted by the great Ming physician and pharmacopoeist Li Shizhen, whom we shall encounter presently.[14] Zhu Quan's several other medical writings are also quoted by Li Shizhen.

Medical writings of the Ming period were already discussing the prevention of smallpox, some two hundred years before Edward Jenner introduced vaccination in England. There is also evidence that vaccination against smallpox had been practised in China since the year 1000 (Needham). Inoculation against smallpox originated in the southwestern province of Sichuan. The Daoist alchemists used the technique in the tenth century AD and practised a variety of methods for the attenuation of the virus so that the chances of getting the disease were minimised and the chances of immunity were maximised. The favourite source of poxy material was the scabs of someone who had been inoculated. The method used was to put the poxy material on some cotton which was then inserted into the nose where it was absorbed through the mucous membrane and by breathing. The general system was to keep the inoculum sample for about a month at body temperature. During the 17th century the practice of inoculation spread to the Turkish region and it was there that it came to the attention of the Europeans. This breakthrough in the treatment of smallpox and its spread to Europe has led to the modern science of immunology.

Let us return very briefly to the compendium of alchemy compiled by the Ming prince Zhu Quan and the pharmacopoeia by his elder half-brother Zhu Su. They both marked a turning point in Chinese alchemy in its relationship with Chinese medicine. As we have noted earlier, many of the early alchemists, such as Ge Hong, Tao Hongjing, Sun Simiao and Meng Shen, were also physicians with great reputation. As we also remember, Chinese medicine was never inhibited by a Galenic doctrine that restricted the physicians in Europe to use medicine only from the vegetable kingdom. In China the physicians and the alchemists used both substances from the vegetable kingdom as well as metals and minerals. In the elixir formulae used by the early Chinese alchemists, such as Ge Hong and Sun Simiao, we find mainly metals and minerals. Of course Ge Hong and Sun Simiao also employed metals and minerals in their medical prescriptions, but the quantity involved was far more conservative than what they used in alchemy. Some of the minerals and metals used by the early alchemists, such as mercury, lead and arsenic, were highly toxic, and consequently many cases of elixir poisoning were reported. A number of Chinese emperors and high officials in medieval China had perished as a result of their ambition to prolong their human lifespan indefinitely. Chinese alchemy must have lost some of its best exponents in this manner, for the most capable were very often the most dedicated and firmest believers, and in the end the surest victims. Chinese alchemists therefore became more cautious in their approach and sought alternative ways and means to attain their objective. One method was to change their elixir ingredients from minerals and metals to plants. Such a change came about around the latter half of the Mongol period when we find writers on alchemy confining their attention to the vegetable kingdom. The pharmacopoeia of Zhu Su and the compendium on alchemy by Zhu Quan represent the last phase when the change from metals and minerals to the vegetable kingdom was more or less completed. It is interesting to note that while Chinese medicine had never been inhibited by the Galenic doctrine on the exclusive use of plant drugs, Chinese alchemy towards its last stages of development came across a similar restriction, imposed not by any orthodox doctrine, but by elixir poisoning, and that Chinese alchemy had rejoined Chinese medicine in the area of plant drugs.

Elixir poisoning may lead some to dismiss alchemy as one of the examples of human follies in history, and in this case, one that was typical of traditional China. But there is one positive aspect of it in its connection with Chinese medicine. The caution given to elixir poisoning also led Chinese alchemy to shade imperceptibly into iatrochemistry, the preparation of medicine by chemical methods, in other words chemotherapy. The medieval Chinese alchemists succeeded in preparing mixtures of androgens and oestrogens in a relatively purified crystalline form and used them in therapy for many hypogonadic conditions. Iatrochemistry, therefore, took root in China many centuries before the time of Paracelsus (1493 to 1541), the "Father of Iatrochemistry" in Europe.

In the 15th century Yang Jizhou wrote the *Zhenjiu daquan* (Compendium of Acupuncture and Moxibustion) (1468) trying to incorporate into it all the existing knowledge on acupuncture. Early in the 16th century the Ming emperor, Xiaozong, ordered Liu Wentai to lead a group of physicians-royal to compile the most comprehensive pharmacopoeia of his time. As a result the *Bencao pinhui jingyao* (The Classified Pharmacopoeia) was published in the year 1505. This official pharmacopoeia was not republished, and as a result it was not available to the general public as well as the medical profession, and hence it has not been given the attention it deserves. In fact the beautiful illustrations in this pharmacopoeia alone are something worthy of attention in the study of illustrations in the early history of botany.

Chinese medicine seems to have reached its peak in the 16th century when Li Shizhen wrote his *Bencao gangmu* (The Great Pharmacopoeia), which describes plants, substances of animal origin, and minerals and metals together with their medical properties and applications. Li Shizhen was born in Hubei province in the year 1518, and was a pharmaceutical naturalist and physician. He began to compile his pharmacopoeia when he was 35 years old and took 27 years in writing it. The text consists of over one million words and it describes in detail 1800 kinds of medicinal plants, among them 300 that had not been cited in previous works. Li Shizhen died in 1593 at the time when the wood blocks for his gigantic work were completed and his book was ready for printing. This pharmacopoeia is a practical guide to medical practice, and discusses such familiar matters as distillation, smallpox immunization and valid therapeutic uses of mercury, sulphur, iodine and kaolin, for example. Needham calls Li Shizhen the greatest naturalist in Chinese history, while Lu Gwei-Djen points out that this great pharmacopoeia turns out to be also a comprehensive treatise on mineralogy, metallurgy, botany and zoology.[15] Li Shizhen's work lists most of the natural medicinal substances used in the Western world today.

The *Bencao gangmu* is perhaps the most influential text in the history of medicine, having been used and later translated by the Koreans and the Japanese. For the Chinese and Koreans it remains the "gospel" in traditional medicine, yet only fragments of it have been translated into English, and those fragments are very difficult to find. Thus, many useful remedies, such as *ephedra*, *rauwolfia* and chaulmoogra were not "discovered" by the West until the 20th century, and many others used quite extensively and effectively by empirical healers are still unfamiliar in "scientific" practice. The latest six-volume edition of the *Bencao gangmu*, available in almost every bookstore in Hong Kong, has been used by more people than any medical book ever written. And this is only one of the many books that form part of the rich Asian medical heritage.

The fact that Asian medical systems were stifled by Western influence, does not reflect upon their essential and lasting value. That does not mean, of course, that today's modern practitioners should abandon their new learning and regress to the level of ancient sages, for even the best old texts are riddled with errors. But neither could they depend today upon the teachings of Pasteur, Lister, or even Osler and other great healers of the 19th and early 20th centuries. Medical science is cumulative, and the achievements of any given period are actually the fruit of all preceding experience. The validity of the achievement depends to a great extent upon how well the innovators have absorbed the lessons of the past.

During the Ming period, Chinese medicine also held sway in Korea, and in Japan where it continued unrivalled until the arrival of the Spanish Jesuit missionary Francis Xavier in the year 1549. Under the Ming and the Qing (1644 to 1911) dynasties social organisations of many kinds decayed, and the hospitals were no exceptions, so that when Westerners began to visit China in any numbers early in the 19th century they gained an entirely wrong picture of the history of medical administration in China. Nevertheless, many interesting hospitals and public charities did continue in those late times.

As mentioned earlier, the Nestorians had already come to China with their medical skill during the 8th century. China's contact with the West, where medicine is concerned, was not appreciable until the arrival of the Jesuits in the late 16th century. The Jesuits introduced some western books on medicine and western knowledge of human anatomy to China. One of the Jesuits, Claudus de Visdelou (1656 to 1737), even cured the Chinese emperor Kangxi of malaria using quinine in the year 1693. However, western medicine then did not have much effect in China and what the Jesuits had written on the subject were merely preserved in the libraries as literary curiosities. For example, even as late as the first quarter of the 19th century, a well-known Qing scholar, Yu Zhengxie, considered that there were basic anatomical and physiological differences between the Europeans and the Chinese, because the anatomical drawings produced by the Jesuits were different from those found in traditional Chinese medical writings. He even went a step further to use this as an argument to prove that Christianity was a religion more suitable to the Europeans than to the Chinese, because the Europeans used the brain while the Chinese used the heart for thinking (that was what traditional Chinese physiology told them).

Since the mid-19th century Western medicine began to reach China in greater number together with Christian missionaries and merchants. It has to be understood that in the Chinese context the term "Western medicine" means the corpus of medical knowledge that had emerged in Western Europe after the Renaissance period (15th and 16th centuries) and which in itself already was an amalgam of practices and ideas that had developed and been diffused by different cultures into the European culture area. One may say that Western medicine was formally introduced into China by Benjamin Hobson (1816 to 1873) with the publication of his works *Xiyi luelun* (Outline of Western Medicine), *Quanti xinbian* (New Anatomy of the Human Body), *Neike xinshuo* (New Discourse on Internal Medicine), and the *Fuying qianshuo* (Simple Discourse on Gynaecology and Paediatrics). A good number of Western medical works were later translated into Chinese by John Fryer (1839 to 1928). Exchange of medical knowledge between Europe and China was not entirely one-sided. Acupuncture, for example, was introduced into Europe by a surgeon employed by the Dutch East India Company, Wilhelm ten Rhyne, whose book on acupuncture, entitled *Dissertatio de Arthritide* was published in London in 1683. In 1712 another Dutchman, Engelbert Kampfer, who was then working in the Dutch Embassy in Japan, published a book in Germany on acupuncture entitled *Avoenitatum Exoticarum*. Both these books received very little attention in Europe. In 1810 acupuncture seems to have been practised for the first time in Europe when a French physician, Louis Berlioz, treated a neurotic patient using this Chinese method and published his results in Paris.

Traditional and Western medicine co-existed for some time in China. However, due to the many differences between the two systems confrontation was the expected outcome. The two distinct advantages of Western medicine over traditional medicine are the orientation of the former to modern science thus becoming what is known as modern medicine, and the more uniform and systematized education that a Western doctor has to go through. However, traditional Chinese medicine contains information extending over a period of two thousand years of past experience, some of which may not yet be known in modern medicine. For example there have been many surprises for pharmacologists in the West in the use of ephedrine from *Ephedra sinica* and *Rauwolfia* with its numerous powerful and peculiar alkaloids from Chinese pharmacopoeias. Unfortunately polarisation developed to the extent of confrontation where Chinese traditional medicine was condemned as being unscientific and regarded as an obstacle to the development of modern medicine in China. By then modern medicine had already been recognised as the official system of medicine in Japan although traditional Chinese medicine in the form of kampō continued to have a following among the Japanese people. In the year 1929 the Chinese government took steps to abolish traditional Chinese medicine. However, strong protests from the public forced the government to back down from its legislation. While modern medicine had become the official system, the practice of traditional medicine continued unabated and has developed to its present stage today.

In 1930 the average lifespan of a person in China was estimated to be 34 years, and by 1995 the estimated life expectancy had increased to 71 years. The crude mortality rate at that time was 25 per thousand while the infant mortality rate was 157 per thousand. These figures worsened during the period from 1940 to 1949 when the crude death rate rose to 30 per thousand and the infant mortality rate to 275 per thousand. The situation began to improve with the attention given to sanitation and medical care after the year 1949. By 1994 the crude mortality rate had dropped to only 6.49 per thousand and the infant mortality rate to 31 per thousand, comparing not unfavourably with a crude mortality rate of 12.1 per thousand and an infant mortality rate of 17.5 per thousand for the same period in England. These figures speak for the remarkable achievements of health workers in China. The above statistics are suggestive of profound improvements in the health of the Chinese people. These achievements are the more remarkable seeing how China has managed to expand rapidly its health care delivery without spending large amounts of money. Traditional medicine has been playing an important role alongside with modern Western medicine in their accomplishment. An interesting example is the small percentage of school children wearing eye-glasses that visitors can observe in China. By carrying out eye exercises based on traditional Chinese medicine for preventing near-sightedness and paying attention to proper lighting in classrooms and correct reading and writing postures, school children in China maintain their good eyesight. This is an example of preventive health care not only at low cost but also with huge savings on the expenditure of providing spectacles. In the late 1980s and 1990s the practice of *qigong*, a traditional system of health and mind control involving deep breathing and other exercises, has undergone an enthusiastic revival.

In 1949 the number of Western-type doctors in China was estimated to be only 20,000 for a population of some 450 million, and the number of traditional doctors was about half a million. Efforts were made to increase the number of these health workers. By 1989 there were 131 medical colleges and 515 medical middle schools. Between 1950 and 1981 some 413,000 medical graduates of western type had been produced, that is, 43.7 times the number that had graduated during the 20 years prior to 1949. And from 1950 to 1981 the medical middle schools had graduated about 940,000 assistant doctors. Also in 1981 there were 20 times more hospital beds than in 1950. On the research side, in 1949 there were four medical research institutes with a staff of less than 300, and in 1981 there were 282 such institutes with a staff of 25,000. In line with the constitutionally specified policy of giving emphasis both to modern and traditional forms of medicine, the government has established a State Traditional Chinese Medicine Administration Bureau under the State Council. In addition, several of the minorities, such as the Tibetans, Mongolians and Uygurs, have their own traditional medicines which are still actively maintained and supported. Of the 1.72 million doctors in China in 1989, 370,000, or 21.5 per cent, were practitioners of traditional Chinese medicine, and there were 22 colleges, 753 hospitals and 47 research institutes. Fully trained doctors were supplemented by rural (barefoot) doctors, all of whom were trained in the rudiments of both Western and traditional medicine. The number of rural doctors in 1977 was estimated to be 1,800,000. Traditional medicine has thus played an important role alongside Western medicine in looking after the health of the Chinese people.

One of the most striking and important characteristics of medicine in China today is the effort to integrate traditional medicine with Western-type medicine. In 1956 Mao Zedong urged these two schools to be integrated so as to create a unified system of medicine. The creation of such a system is considered to be one of the important goals in China's attempt to modernise science and technology by the end of this century.

In China today traditional doctors are working alongside Western-type doctors in hospitals, medical schools and research institutes. This also applies to traditional native doctors in places like Inner Mongolia and Tibet, where attention is given to the traditional medicine of the Minorities. At first, doctors of the two schools only held consultations among themselves, or a Western-type doctor would make the diagnosis and a traditional doctor would give the treatment, depending on the case itself. The result of the treatment was to be observed by both. Gradually the two schools learned to work together in diagnosis, treatment, observations and case summary. Some of the Western-type doctors who were initially reluctant to accept the traditional system of medicine, have now been won over after witnessing the results achieved. Students studying Western-type medicine have now to study traditional medicine for one or two years, and special handbooks on traditional medicine have been written for them.

One of the centres noted for its effort to integrate traditional Chinese medicine with Western medicine is the Nankai Hospital in Tianjin. Nevertheless we can find similar efforts being made in many other hospitals all over China. In the Hongkou Central Hospital in Shanghai and also in a small hospital in the Changqing Commune in Suzhou, which one of us (Ho) visited with a group of students from Griffith University in December 1978, one can have the opportunity to observe the combined practice of the two schools of medicine in China today.

Medical workers in China have found that the combination of traditional Chinese medicine and modern Western medicine is not only often simpler and more economical but can also produce better and quicker results. One example is the treatment of chronic bronchitis, which is quite common in China. Through chemical analysis and animal tests of different herbs used in various parts of China in traditional medicine for the treatment of coughs and asthma Chinese medical workers have produced a new medicine, *Vitex cannabifolia volatile*, which has proved effective for the treatment of chronic bronchitis as well as in the reduction of the incidence of pulmonary emphysema and pulmonary heart disease.

Another example is the use of traditional Chinese herbs for the treatment of severe burns. Since 1969 Chinese medical workers have been studying the use of *Ilex chinensis* for this purpose. They found that this plant contains a large quantity of tannin, which induces scab formation and inhibits the growth of *Bacillus pyocyaneus* and *Staphlococcus aureus*, often associated with burn infections. In the past the tannin from *alla sinensis* used clinically for treating burns was found to be toxic to the liver, giving rise to acute necrosis, and was thus discontinued during the 1940's. *Ilex chinensis,* however, does not seem to cause jaundice or do any noticeable harm to the liver, even in cases where the burns cover more than half the body. With *Ilex chinensis* most cases of burns in China can now be treated in ordinary clinics without modern facilities and with far fewer dressings, simpler nursing care and lower costs.

In China traditional medicine also plays an important role in the fight against cancer. By the combined use of traditional medicine and Western medicine, Chinese medical workers attack the disease by surgery, radiation, and chemotherapy, and build up the patient's resistance by the administration of herbal medicine. A number of Chinese herbs have been found effective under certain conditions, and many anti-cancer drugs have been produced in China. It has been reported that the bark, root and fruits of *Camptotheca acuminata*, Decne, for example, have been found effective in the treatment of leukemia and cancer of the stomach, liver and bladder. In June 1978 Dr Henry Ekert, the Director of the Clinical Haematology and Oncology Department at Melbourne Royal Children's Hospital, was reported to have spoken about a Chinese drug very effective in the treatment of acute leukemia, called Harringtonine, which is an extract from the *Cephalotaxus hainanensis* li. tree.[16] The leaves of the *Cycas revoluta*, Thunb. tree have also been found effective for the treatment of cancer of the liver according to another report.

Combined use of traditional medicine and Western medicine has eliminated the necessity of surgery in certain cases. One report concerns the successful removal of gallstones under 4 cm in diameter with herbal medicine. It is said that 82 per cent of the over 600 patients with gallstones in the common bile duct admitted to the Qingdao Hospital in Shandong province during the past few years, succeeded in having their stones removed without surgery. Acute abdominal diseases have also been successfully treated by the combined use of traditional medicine and Western medicine. In the four years before 1978 some 80 per cent of the 2000 acute abdominal cases in Nankai Hospital were treated by such methods without surgery, with a reported mortality rate of only 1.2 percent. Another reported example can be found in the treatment of prolapse of the anus due to haemorrhoids and fistula. Surgery would sometimes result in anal stricture, particularly in complex fistulas. Quicker and more effective results have been obtained by adopting the traditional Chinese method of thread therapy.

Traditional Chinese medicine is particularly strong in orthopaedics. Combination of traditional and Western medicine has brought about a new method in the treatment of fractures in China. In the treatment of fractures of the limbs, Western medicine advocates the immobilisation of the limb in plaster after a fracture has been reduced, and if the fracture cannot be reduced or the reduction is unstable, then the patient has to be operated on and the fracture has to be fixed by means of stainless steel plates and screws. Some patients suffer bedsores or stiffening of the joints because of prolonged immobilisation and traction. The new method takes a leaf from traditional medicine by using small splints instead of plaster. It has succeeded in speeding up the healing process. For example, a fracture of the femur, which normally takes about 85 days to heal when treated by modern Western methods, has been reported to take only 52 days under the combined method.

The outside world has heard much more about acupuncture than any other aspects of traditional Chinese medicine. In the 1960's China astonished the outside world by reports a nd photographs of patients in hospitals undergoing operations, while fully conscious, through the use of acupuncture analgesia. Hundreds of thousands of cases of operations, including the removal of brain tumours, opening the chest and caesarean sections, performed under acupuncture analgesia have been reported. Towards the end of 1976 acupuncture analgesia was used in all obstetrical and gynaecological operations in a Shanghai hospital. The acupuncture point for this purpose lies below the spinous process of the eleventh thoracic vertebra. The same point is now also used in gastrectomy and for the removal of various abdominal tumours in some Chinese hospitals. In 1977 one of us (Lisowski) witnessed the use of acupuncture analgesia at a Zhengzhou hospital in cases of thyroidectomy, lobectomy (removal of part of the lung) and hysterectomy, and in December 1978, one of us (Ho) witnessed two operations using this technique, one for thyroidectomy and one for hernia repair in the Hongkou Central Hospital in Shanghai, and was informed by the superintendent of that hospital that every anaesthetist providing acupuncture analgesia was a fully trained Western-type anaesthetist, and could easily change to the conventional type of analgesia if conditions warranted. The superintendent, himself a Western-type doctor, also said that patients undergoing operations were given a choice between acupuncture and Western-type analgesia. The Chinese are fully aware of the fact that acupuncture analgesia is not a foolproof method of analgesia and that it works only for certain types of patients.

The use of acupuncture to block pain has a history of only three decades. The other aspect of acupuncture, its general use for therapeutic purposes, has also made notable progress. Acupuncture is now being practised within and outside China in many forms of neuritic and spasmodic pains, such as painful disorders of the musculoskeletal system, lumbago, neuralgias, shingles, pains in amputation stumps, dysmenorrhoea and various colics and post-traumatic pains, not to mention rheumatism and arthritis. It is also used to treat cases of digestive disorder, allergic diseases like asthma and eczema, cardiovascular complaints like tachycardia, extrasystoles, hypertension, hypotension, and arteritis, enuresis and withdrawal symptoms in drug addicts, and also impetigo and varicose ulcers. It also gives good results in cases of depression, worry and insomnia. In 1978 two cases of acupuncture treatment, one for arthritis and the other for dysmenorrhoea, performed at the Hongkou Central Hospital in Shanghai and a case of lumbago treatment performed at a commune hospital near Suzhou were also observed.

In China traditional doctors and Western-type doctors still talk different languages, professionally speaking. The former use terms like *Yin* and *Yang* and talk about acupuncture points and tracts, for which the Western-type doctors can find no anatomical basis so far. We are reminded of a lecture given by Joseph Needham in 1967 at the Leeds Meeting of the British Association.[17] At that meeting he pointed out that the physical sciences like mathematics, astronomy and physics of West and East united very quickly after they first came together. By 1644, the end of the Ming dynasty, there was no longer any perceptible difference between the mathematics, astronomy and physics of

China and Europe. The biological sciences took longer to fuse. In botany, for example, it was not until 1880 that fusion took place. However, the coming together of the two cultural traditions of Chinese and modern Western medicine, the fusion into one unitary modern medical science, has not yet been effected. With the great effort made in China nowadays to encourage the study of traditional medicine, to integrate traditional Chinese with modern Western medicine, and with the dispassionate scientific research carried out both inside and outside China, for example on acupuncture, the day when the two traditions fuse promises to be closer at hand than Needham foresaw in 1967.

We would expect that most of the new contributions to medical science coming from China in the near future will be the results of integrating traditional and modern Western medicine. An abundant supply of water will be brought along by the long river of traditional Chinese medicine when it joins the ocean of modern medicine, and modern medicine is likely to be enriched through research on traditional medicine in China. Perhaps the Chinese model can serve as a good reference for other traditional medicines in Asia. We are referring especially to West Asian and South Asian traditional medicine and wish to express our hope that they too will play their part and add to the knowledge of modern medicine.

Perhaps the most difficult hurdle to overcome lies in the difficulty for the traditional Chinese concept of the art of healing to find acceptance in modern medicine. We would like to conclude this account with a view of modern medicine *vis a vis* its Chinese counterpart taken from the standpoint of traditional Chinese concepts. Modern medicine employs modern science both as a tool for patient care and in its attempts to explain its methods, and thus in terms of modern science it is much "clearer" to understand and more "positive" than the Chinese traditional art of healing. Modern medicine uses chemical products which are generally more "potent" but also with more side-effects than the herbs normally used in Chinese medicine, and at the same time the action of the former is more "direct". In terms of their organisation that of modern medicine is far more "active" and "assertive" than that of the latter. Modern medicine can thus be seen as possessing all the qualities of the *Yang* as compared to the traditional Chinese healing art which has to be regarded in this case as *Yin*. *Yin* and *Yang* are always opposite and yet they always co-exist and are complementary to each other. The Chinese traditional art of healing, practised today along side with modern medicine, not only in China but also in Korea and Japan albeit in a modified form, seems to have a future whichever way one looks at it.

Notes

1. A full treatment of the whole subject will be given in Joseph Needham, *Science and Civilisation in China*, Vol. 6, parts 7 to 10 (Institutes of Medicine, Medicine, Pharmaceutics); meanwhile see Joseph Needham, *Clerks and Craftsmen in China and the West*, Cambridge University Press, 1970 and Joseph Needham (with Lu Gwei-Djen), *Celestial Lancets: A History and Rationale of Acupuncture and Moxa*, Cambridge University Press, 1980. Active research on the theory of Chinese medicine is being pursued by a number of other scholars, for example, Nathan Sivin of the University of Pennsylvania. Meanwhile much research on the subject of traditional medicine is being carried out in China, principally at the Institute of Traditional Chinese Medicine, Beijing.

2. See, for example, Beijing Chinese College of Chinese Medicine, *Zhongguo yixueshi jiangyi*, Hong Kong, 1968, p. 3.

3. For a full translation of the *Suwen* see, for example, Veith, I., *Huang-ti nei ching su wen* (The Yellow Emperor's Classic of Internal Medicine), Berkeley, 1972, and for a description of this book given by a Cambridge-trained M.D. of Chinese origin with the collaboration of another Western-trained Chinese physician, see Wu Lien-teh and Wang Chi-min, *History of Chinese Medicine*, Shanghai, 1932, 2nd edition 1936, pp. 28 ff.

4. We are indebted to our friend Dr Janet Fowler for Figs. 1 and 2.

5. For a Western view on the theory of Chinese medicine see, for example, M. Porkert, *The Theoretical Foundation of Chinese Medicine*, Cambridge, Mass. 1974. Porkert much prefers "the Five Phases" to "the Five Elements".

6. Nowadays traditional Chinese practitioners speak also in terms of the "main medicine" for combating the source of illness, "adjunct medicine" that assists the "main medicine", "harmonizing medicine" that produces

a happy mixture of the various ingredients in a medical prescription, and "guiding medicine" that leads the "main medicine" to the site of the illness. See, for example, *Xinbian zhongyixue gaiyao*, Beijing, 1972, 3rd ed., 1974, pp. 149–150.

7. See Saburô Miyashita, "A Neglected Source for the Early History of Anaesthesia in China and Japan", In Shigeru Nakayama and Nathan Sivin, eds., *Chinese Science: Exploration of an Ancient Tradition*, Cambridge, Mass. 1973, p. 273.

8. Gwee Ah Leng, *Medicine East and West: A direct Comparison*, Singapore, 1968, pp. 26–29 describes the technique of pulse-reading from the standpoint of a Western-trained M.D. who came from the family of a traditional Chinese physician.

9. Some examples from this medical treatise are given in W.C. Cooper and Nathan Sivin, "Man as a medicine: Pharmacological and Ritual Aspects of Traditional Therapy using Drugs derived from the Human Body", In Shigeru Nakayama and Nathan Sivin, eds., *Chinese Science: Exploration of an Ancient Tradition*, Cambridge, Mass., 1973, pp. 203–272. This text shows some early traces of Indian medicine which came to China in the wake of Buddhism.

10. Some of the medicinal herbs that went from China to Japan during the Tang period are still preserved in the Shôsôin. See Asahina Yasuhiko et al, *Shôsôin yakubutsu*, Osaka, 1955. Hakim Mohamed Said, "Medieval Chinese, Japanese and Arab medicine: Reciprocal impact", *Hamdard Medicus*, Vol. 19, 1976, pp. 99–109 has more to say about intercultural contacts.

11. His *Taiqing danjing yaojue* is fully translated in Nathan Sivin, *Chinese Alchemy: Preliminary Studies*, Cambridge, Mass., 1968.

12. For an English version see Giles, H.A., "The *Hsi Yuan Lu* or Instructions to Coroners", *Pro. Roy. Soc. Med.* Vol. 17, 1924, pp. 59 ff. One interesting example in this book is the use of a hen as a test-animal in forensic medicine. Se Ho, P.Y. and Needham, J., "Elixir Poisoning in Medieval China", *Janus*, Vol. 47, 1959, pp. 221–251.

13. This pharmacopoeia was a topic of an M. Phil. dissertation by Chan Yuet Ling at the Department of Chinese, University of Hong Kong in 1985.

14. See Ho Peng Yoke and Chiu Ling Yeong, *Ningwang Zhu Quan jiqi Gengxin yuce*, Hong Kong, 1983.

15. See Lu Gwei-Djen, "China's great naturalist: A brief biography of Li Shih-chen", *Physis, Rivista Internazionale di storia della scienza*, Vol. 8, 1966, pp. 383–392.

16. An interview with Dr Henry Ekert, Director of the Clinical Haematology and Oncology Department at Melbourne Royal Children's Hospital, reported in the *Courier-Mail* (23rd June 1978), p. 10.

17. See Joseph Needham, "The Roles of Europe and China in the Evolution of Oecumenical Sciences", *Advancement of Science*, Sept.1967, pp. 87–98.

Part 2

AREAS INFLUENCED BY CHINESE THOUGHT

Part 2

AREAS INFLUENCED BY CHINESE THOUGHT

Chinese medical concepts and practice had a profound influence on the neighbouring countries of East, Southeast and South Asia. They also penetrated westwards along the ancient Silk Road to Persia and thereby became absorbed into the Arab world. Between China and India there were reciprocal influences, along the trade routes through Burma in the east and the Khunjerab Pass in the Karakoram mountain range in the west.

We cite two examples in our account of Chinese thought penetration, one where there was a profound influence, namely Japan, and one which the eddies of Chinese medical thought touched, namely the Islamic world.

A BRIEF HISTORY OF MEDICINE IN JAPAN

Historically Japan grew up within a cultural environment in eastern Asia in which China was the centre. However, the isolation of the Japanese islands has made for an unusually unified and self-contained history. Protected from the play of competing civilisations or the periodic disruption of foreign invasion, the Japanese people in historic times have lived a relatively undisturbed existence. Yet their culture has undergone a succession of fundamental changes that transformed it from a primitive tribal society prior to the sixth century into a nation of aristocratic bureaucrats from the seventh through the twelfth centuries; later, into a land of contending feudal powers; and finally, into its present condition as a modern nation state.

Japan's position on the extreme fringes of the Chinese zone of civilisation has made it possible for her people, through absorbing Chinese culture in great quantity, to yet retain a firm hold on their own feudal institutions, its maritime orientation and its strong sense of nationality.

The Japanese people have escaped the experience of devastating foreign invasions. Throughout their premodern history, structural changes have come slowly and have been brought about more by internal forces than external pressures.

From about 7000 to 250 BC (the Jōmon culture) the people of these islands were food gatherers, hunters and fishermen. This period was followed by the Yayoi culture which was the beginning of the agricultural era. Gradually a peasant base was formed which was characterised by a high ratio of cultivators to units of land, and a high ratio of agricultural production to that of the total economy. This was made possible through a highly sophisticated system of water control and village and family organisation. The peasant base remained rooted to the soil and preoccupied with the problems of land and water.

It was in this environment that early indigenous Japanese medicine developed. Evidence of healed fractures, trepanations of skulls and other findings of those times indicate that some form of medical practice must have existed. During the fourth to sixth centuries AD Chinese medicine was introduced by way of Korea. In the year 414 the Korean physician Kim Mu arrived in Japan. This was the first authenticated contact with Korean medicine. And in 456 a Korean physician by the name of Doklei established himself in Naniwa (Osaka).

In 561 a Japanese general, pursuing a military campaign in Korea, sent a physician, Zhicong, who came from central China, to Japan. The latter brought with him 164 books on medicine, surgery, herbal medicine and an atlas of acupuncture and moxibustion.

Several large epidemics of plague and smallpox ravaged the country between the third and eight centuries. These had entered Japan from Korea.

During the middle of the sixth century Buddhism came to Japan by way of Korea. This had a profound influence on the whole subsequent history of the culture of the country.

In the seventh century official and private interchanges between China and Japan flourished, and a large number of Japanese students travelled to China in order to study. On the other hand, owing to the political turmoil of the time in Korea, many artisans and scientists emigrated to Japan to augment the local forces to the benefit of the host country.

During the Nara period (702 to 783), in the year 710, Nara became the capital of Japan with an architectural style and a system of administration based on that of Tang China. A hospital and a dispensary were established in 730, the first of such institutions in Japan, as well as a government medical system: The Office of Medical Authority (Tenyakuryo) which was responsible for the supervision and provision of medical assistance in the capital. This office was also concerned with the training of students in the craft of acupuncture and moxibustion, herbal medicine, and pulse diagnosis. The training was based on the study of Chinese texts. The Office provided specialist courses in internal medicine (six years), surgery (five years), paediatrics (five years), ear-nose-and-throat diseases (four years), dentistry (four years), and acupuncture and moxibustion (six years). Students who had not passed their examinations within nine years had to withdraw from the course.

The medical system and the study of medicine during the Nara period were a copy of the system prevailing in China of the Tang dynasty. The concept of the pathology of disease was also that current in China at that time; alongside this, indigenous thought attributed the causal factors to malign deities.

The treatment at that time consisted principally of diet therapy, medicines prepared from herbal, animal and mineral substances, rice wine, acupuncture, moxibustion and hydrotherapy. A number of texts on therapy were produced as well as books on herbal medicine, most of these came from China. In one of the texts of c.757 first mention is made of medicaments from India.

Of special interest are the allusions to anatomical dissection during the fifth century. A chronicle of the year 454 describes how a young princess who had committed suicide underwent an autopsy. Some years later observations were made on a human fetus. Subsequently an embargo was placed on these procedures and no further references to dissection are found in the historical accounts of Japanese medicine.

Accounts of the high mortality rate during outbreaks of typhus are given, and there are descriptions of typhoid, smallpox, dysentery and other diseases.

During the Heian period (784 to 1192) the capital moved from Nara to Kyoto. The model of China was gradually abandoned and an indigenous system began to show itself which was reflected particularly in the central administration. Chinese civilisation had by now been assimilated beyond the point of conscious imitation. There was evidence of a noticeable assimilation of Buddhist beliefs. This had penetrated the common religious beliefs of the Japanese and became fused with Shinto shrine worship. By Heian times the Buddhist priesthood had taken over administration of a sizeable number of local shrines.

The aristocracy, living in unhygienic conditions, were very much concerned with immortality. One of the principal functions of the physicians of that time was to prescribe medical preparations that helped to prolong life. Thus various elixirs such as concoctions and pills composed of tin, lead, mercury and gold were prescribed. The application of these metallic compounds had originated with the Taoists in China.

An important work, the *Ishino* of thirty volumes, was produced by a court physician, Yasuyori Tamba (912 to 995). This was in many ways a copy of the *Zhubingyuan haolun* (Treatise on the Origins and Symptoms of Disease) by Chao Yuanfang of the early Tang period in China. Tamba referred to various Chinese texts and possibly encountered references to Indian and Arabic medicine. The *Ishino* continued to be of such importance that its original text was still consulted in the 16th century.

The Heian period also saw a great increase in the production of Japanese medical books. This was a result of the rise in nationalism, a reaction to the previous dominance of the Tang culture, which in turn gave rise to a revaluation of indigenous medicine. During this period too, various epidemics such as smallpox, influenza and parotitis swept through Japan.

In 1192 the administrative bureaucracy gave way to the feudal system. There was a breakup of the monopoly of power held since the eighth century by the court-based aristocracy and the central monasteries. At the same time new institutions of political authority and land control appeared. All this contributed to the abolition of state medicine, though it persisted in at least a nominal form. The state medical service which had been established in the eighth century was unable to satisfy the real needs. As a result a new type of physician made his appearance, the medical priest who was more or less a private practitioner.

During the twelfth to fourteenth centuries Buddhism became a popular religion. This was particularly so owing to the decadence of the rulers, the corruption and disorder of the times. Monasteries were established and physician priests practised among the population. The first medical texts in the Japanese language and a variety of medical schools (ryū) appeared. A national consciousness began to develop.

Eisai (1141 to 1215) was a physician priest and the founder of the Zen sect. His *Kissa Yōjyōki* (Treatise on the Medical Use of Tea) recommended the discipline of Buddhism and the harmonious function of the internal organs through careful selection of food. Eisai advised that infusions of tea maintained the health of the body.

According to the ancient law, Taiho Codes (701), medicine was classified into tairyō (internal medicine) and sōshu (surgery). Later in the twelfth century the former was called hondō and the latter geka. Although there were professional surgeons at that time, there were no real books on surgery and the actual surgical treatment differed little from that performed by the physician.

Surgeons were further divided into yōka or furuncle surgeons who specialised in incising furuncles and boils and kinsōi or wound surgeons who specialised in the treatment of sword wounds inflicted on the battlefield. Many kinsōi also acted as obstetricians.

The relationship between the yōka and kinsōi seems to have been similar to that between the chirurgien-barbier (surgeon-barber) and barbier-chirurgien (barber-surgeon) during the Renaissance period in France. The kinsōi physicians tended to look down on and to humiliate the surgeons because most of the latter's work was considered messy and dirty. Actually many of those who practised surgery at that time were illiterate, similar to the barbier-chirurgien in France.

Seigan (? to 1379) was the first known ophthalmologist so far in the world. He was a priest and the founder of the Majima sect. This sect specialised in the treatment of eye diseases. The treatment consisted in the main of internal medication, lotions, the application of ointments and powders, vapours, diets and operations. The operative procedures consisted of cauterisation and the use of lancets, the latter use being a secret procedure reputed to have been applied in the removal of cataract.

During the Song period relations with China were interrupted and Japan entered a difficult time of division and civil wars which impeded cultural development. Orthodox medicine and the activity of the priest physicians went into decline.

With the flowering of the Ming dynasty, Japan renewed her contacts with China, and many students went there to study medicine, often staying for one or two decades.

Syōkei Takeda went to China in 1365 and Gekko in 1444; both published numerous treatises on their return. And Sanki Tashiro (1465 to 1537), another returned student, taught Dōsan Manase (1506 to 1594) who restored medicine to its former eminence in Japan and also founded a school of medicine.

There was a revaluation of classical medicine and various schools arose and contended. Two main rival factions arose: one, the Gose-ha, which accepted the theories of Ming medicine, and the other, the kohōha, which maintained the classical Chinese view.

The decline of Buddhist doctrine and of related medical literature towards the end of the 16th century can be attributed to the introduction of Ming medicine. This brought about a renaissance in acupuncture and moxibustion, and the detailed study of the pulse for diagnostic purposes.

In 1543 a Portuguese ship drifted ashore at the southern end of Japan during a typhoon. This incident was the first direct encounter with western Europe. And in 1556 a Portuguese surgeon, Louis de Almeida (1525 to 1584), arrived in Japan with a group of missionaries.

Western medical care was at first practised for the purpose of spreading the Christian religion. The earliest centres were established in Osaka, Sakai and Nagasaki. The practice in these places continued even after missionary work had been suppressed. The new type of surgery that had been introduced was called Namban surgery. Namban means "southern barbarian" because the practice came from the "southern sea". Many books of this period were dictated handwritten notes which were often incomplete.

Following the prohibition of missionary work, the Spanish were expelled in 1624 and the Portuguese in 1639. As a result their trade ceased. The Tokugawa government (1603 to 1867) adopted a closed-country policy, being especially strict on missionary activity and religious literature. However, the Dutch were allowed to continue their trade since they did not engage in or attempt to spread the Christian religion.

Gradually Dutch physicians began to transmit western medicine. Those who wished to study medicine came to Nagasaki from all over Japan where it was taught by the Dutch through Japanese interpreters. The culture which entered Japan through the Dutch language was called Kōmō culture (Kōmō means red hair). Thus it came about that Dutch medicine was best understood by a select group of Japanese interpreters.

It is interesting to note that only surgery was extensively adopted while other branches of medicine were neglected. This is probably because it was possible to demonstrate surgical techniques thereby facilitating a visual understanding, thus overcoming the language barrier. Furthermore, it is remarkable that interpreters, who were not related to medicine, rather than those who came to study the subject, propagated medical practice, each interpreter in due course representing his own school of surgery. In a very short time interpreter-surgeons who understood surgery in words rather than in practice became prominent experts on the subject. These practitioners had a high social standing because of the good effect of their treatment. They obtained high positions which the kinsōi never did. During the Edo era four vertical social classes had been fixed: warriors, farmers, craftsmen and traders. Physicians, along with priests, were outside this system, they were considered as a special group. They had shaved heads and wore a special costume called jittoku.

Of course alongside these developments the traditional practice continued. Whenever Confucianism gained in influence, as during the 17th century, the study of orthodox traditional Chinese medicine advanced and other developments in medicine declined, while a decline in Confucianism tended to stimulate new ideas and advances.

Among some of the earlier well-known interpreter-surgeons was Chinzan Narabayashi (1648 to 1711). He was born in Nagasaki and became an interpreter at the age of 19. He interpreted for and thereby learnt surgery from a Dutch physician, Hoffman, who was attached to the trade centre and who had come to Japan in 1671. In 1678 Narabayashi resigned from this position as interpreter and devoted himself to Kōmō surgery. In 1706 he completed a translation of part of the textbook of surgery by Ambroise Paré (1510 to 1590), the French surgeon. This was the *Kōigeka-Sōden*. The work included what Narabayashi had learnt from different Dutch physicians as well as from his own experience. The book, though never printed, was transmitted in written form. Paré's textbook of surgery had been translated into Dutch by Carolus Battus and had been published in Dordrecht in 1649. It is from this edition that Narabayashi produced his work. However, the latter never mentioned anywhere in his text the author or Dutch translator or indeed anything about the source. This is understandable since at that time even the interpreters were not allowed to read Dutch books; they could only make notes from verbal translations. Permission to import Dutch texts was first granted in 1720. Although the Kōigeka-Sōden is only a partial translation, it does represent the first translation of a western medical book into Japanese.

Narabayashi was a prominent surgeon of his time and yet never employed by the government. He had many pupils and some of his descendants became well-known surgeons. His group was called the Narabayashi School.

Subsequently Latin, German, English and the original French editions of Paré entered Japan.

By the 18th century it is clear that Japan had entered a new phase of urban-centred commercial economy. Urban growth had been astounding. Edo (later Tokyo) had acquired a population of a million, certainly more than contemporary London or Paris. Thus the trend away from agriculture began. Transportation and communication facilities also increased. There was also a rapid development of a currency and exchange system.

In order to maintain the feudal system the Edo government continued the closed-country policy. But public pressure, in particular from the trading section, favouring the opening of Japan to foreign trade mounted. However, the government issued laws prohibiting Dutch science and thus pressure was also exerted on medicine. In addition political manoeuvres by physicians, who tried to protect traditional medical practice, helped to suppress Western medicine for some time. Surgery and ophthalmology, however, were not included among the prohibitions. As a result Western-type surgery acquired a firm position, finally becoming an equal partner of medicine.

In 1765 the first official school of Chinese medicine was founded in Edo.

Dissection of the human cadaver, the study of anatomy, only began in the latter half of the 18th century in Japan. In 1754 the first dissection took place. Gempaku Sugita (1733 to 1817), an interpreter-surgeon, observed a dissection of an executed criminal in 1771 in Edo and was surprised by the accuracy of the anatomical description of the Dutch texts. He translated the work of J.A. Kulmus, commonly known as *Tafel Anatomia* which was published as the *Kaitai Shinsho*. This translation spread widely and informed the Japanese physicians how European medicine of that time viewed the structure-function relationships of the human body. An important development that began to penetrate Japanese medicine at that stage was that the translations were beginning to be influenced by the experience of Japanese physicians. No longer did they rely on translations pure and simple. It is said that Europeanisation of Japanese medicine dates from 1771. Between 1770 and 1860 some 1500 Dutch medical books were translated.

Shingen Kagawa (1702 to 1777) was one of the early physicians who in 1765 described the normal fetal position in the uterus. This was fourteen years after William Smellie, the London obstetrician, had published his observations. Kagawa had learnt obstetrics on his own and had made several original technical innovations, such as the delivery forceps and the method of extraction of the fetus. He published his work in a unique text called *Sanron* (Treatise of Obstetrics).

Interesting observations were made on renal function in experimental studies of animals by Soteki Fuseya (1747 to 1811) and his collaborators. They put forward a theory of filtration in the formation of urine in 1806. This was thirty-six years prior to the well-known work of W. Bowman of London in 1842.

General anaesthesia was discovered in Japan by Seishū Hanaoka (1760 to 1835), the son of a surgeon. After studying in Kyoto he returned to Kishu to practise. As a result the Hanaoka school of surgery became quite famous. The general anaesthetic, Mafutsu-san or Tsūsen-san consisted of six crude drugs of which the main constituent was *Datura alba Nees*, a powerful narcotic. On the 13th of October, 1805 Hanaoka used the anaesthetic for the first time when successfully removing a breast cancer in a 60-year old woman.

Smallpox was a constant scourge in Japan. As Dutch medicine spread, the practice of vaccination, which had entered the country in 1848, began to gain favour.

For Japan a gathering foreign crisis began to appear. The new European societies were the product of the 18th century wars of consolidation which forged a new style of nation state; they were the product of social revolution which forced the individual into closer participation with national life, including universal military service; they were the products of revolutions which came in the wake of the Protestant Reformation and the growth of rationalistic, scientific thought; and they were the products of an economic revolution marked by the growth of industry and science. By the outbreak of the French Revolution in 1789 Europe was on the verge of an explosion which was to carry it across the globe in a wave of expansion and colonisation.

In the 19th century both China and Japan had to face a major national crisis. Both countries were confronted with increasing Western pressure and as a result underwent considerable turmoil. The initial Tokugawa seclusion policy had been enacted against the old colonial powers and had been maintained with little difficulty for well over a century. But by the end of the 18th century, the Japanese were forced to realise that the outside world had changed. The new European and American powers were preparing to break down Japan's walls of isolation. The first pressure came from the north, from Russia. The southern thrust was mounted by Britain: she was concentrating on China and that gave Japan momentary relief from direct British pressure. Thus it happened that it was the eastern thrust coming from the United States that forced Japan to open her doors to foreign trade and an alien culture.

In China and Japan the old political structure was broken and long entrenched vested interests were weakened. In both countries modernisation was closely associated with political revolution against the old regime. This brought about unrest and dislocation in the very fabric of their socioeconomic systems of the time. Technological change and industrial growth were essential if they were to survive economically. The speed with which Japan met these challenges was remarkable, though of course it also brought about considerable turmoil in the country. The new leadership which seized power in 1868 proceeded to create a unified nation state and to enact fundamental reforms calculated to put Japan on the road to rapid modernisation. These events are known as the Meiji Restoration. The new imperial government transferred its operations in 1868 from Kyoto to Edo; the latter was renamed Tokyo. That was also a decisive turning point when the Japanese embargo on foreign influence came to an end.

In 1861 the first official Western-type medical schools were founded in Edo and Nagasaki. The latter was under the direction of Pompe van Meedervoort, a medical officer with a Dutch trading company.

Following the decision to adopt Western technology, the government considered the situation in science and medicine and decided to adopt German medicine as the model in place of the Dutch version. In the spring of 1871 two German military surgeons, Leopold Müller and Theodore Hoffmann came to take charge of the precursor and later Faculty of Medicine of the University of Tokyo. German then became the language of science and medicine in Japan, and medical schools were organised along German lines. Their medical graduates were sent all over the country to different institutions and hospitals as teachers and practitioners.

After 1945 the influence in the medical sciences came more from America. Ever since the middle of the last century, however, there has been a growing indigenous development so that today one can say Japan stands together in the forefront of medical research with other advanced countries.

A BRIEF NOTE ON THE HISTORY OF MEDICINE IN THE ISLAMIC WORLD

After the death of the prophet Muhammad in 632 and the defeat of the tribes of central Arabia which had revolted against Islam, the unparalleled expansion of the Arabs took place. Within a century they had created an empire stretching from the Indian border to the Atlantic coasts of Spain and north Africa, with its main centres in Persia, Syria and Egypt. Countries had fallen to the Arabs whose population had reached a high level of culture, which was deeply influenced by Greek ideas and thus in certain areas presented a relatively uniform development.

Before this conquest western Asia had become more and more christianised, and as a result the Greek language lost its significance in this area as the lingua franca, while the local languages flourished again. Since intellectuals and scholars no longer always understood Greek, the need became apparent to translate the Greek works into the national languages. However, only medical texts and those of the natural sciences were translated since these were considered useful then for the lifestyle. Thus after the conquest, the Arabs could only acquire that part of the Greek corpus of learning which the Syrians and Egyptians were then in a position to offer.

The medicine of the world of Islam, Arabic medicine, therefore was at first largely based on the influence of Greek civilisation. It has to be noted that when cultures meet and manifest themselves in great translating activity, it is customary to differentiate between two phases: one of reception, and one of assimilation. In the phase of reception, which precedes in time, foreign books are at first only translated; later, in the phase of assimilation, the translated texts themselves are independently worked into new books. Of course at times reception and assimilation may also occur at the same time. Before the year 800, translations were few and scanty but after that Greek works were received in profusion.

Of all the Greek physicians, Galen (c.AD 129 to 199) was for the Arabs by far the most significant. His teachings greatly influenced Arabic medicine; these included his theories on the humours, the physiology of metabolism, the three digestions and the movement of the blood. From Galen comes the conception of the four effective grades of medicines and the teleological thinking that seeks to recognise and explain each organ and each natural process in terms of its purpose. Since the third century his medicine had dominated the eastern Mediterranean area. By the second half of the ninth century nearly all of Galen's works had been translated into Arabic. Thus it was that his teachings largely determined Arabic medicine in all essential points. He provided also the rationalism that has left its impression on most Arabic writings.

The tradition of Hippocrates only followed in the shadow of Galen, though the name of Hippocrates was indeed also famous among the Arabs. The fact that the Hippocratic Oath was demanded from the Arab doctors shows how strongly and for how long medical ethics was tied to his name.

Arabic pharmacology received its strongest impulse through the *Materia medica* of Dioscurides (written c.AD 77) of which not only the five original books but also the apocryphal books vi and vii on poisonous plants and animals were translated. In a similar way the texts of many other Greek physicians were translated.

Although the Syrians did translate many works directly from Greek, or from Syrian, into Arabic, they did not confine themselves purely to the role of mediator. Being conversant with the concepts and contents of Greek medicine, they had published independent writings in their own language which were then translated in the ninth century into Arabic. The lines of transmission that led from Greece through Persia to the Arabs were similar to those in the Syrian region. Because of the favoured geographical position, Persia took much from Indian and somewhat less from Chinese medicine.

As one can see, the Arabs were influenced from five sides: by the Greeks, Syrians, Persians, Indians, and the Chinese. In this, the role of transmitting the Greek, Indian, or Chinese legacy fell chiefly to the Syrians and Persians. The Chinese influence came overland by way of the Silk Road and by sea from southern China.

The historical period of Arabic medicine, which lasted more than seven centuries, coincided with the most flourishing period of Islam. Arabic medicine offers therefore a very colourful and varied history. There was no lack of outside stimulus, and one wonders whether this might not have led to a lively argument with Galenism, and whether Galen's doctrine might not have been severely tested or even revised. There were indeed some cases in which individual doctrines of Galen were criticised, but there was no revision, far less dissolution, of the general Galenic system.

The medical crafts of the Arabs and the Persians also served as an example to the world, reaching new heights under al-Rāzī (Rhazes) (AD 850 to 925) and Ibn Sīnā (Avicenna) (AD 980 to 1037), and there is historical evidence that both had been influenced by Chinese and Ayurvedic learning. In the year AD 931, the first qualifying examinations took place under a decree by the Caliph al-Muqtadir in Baghdad. This has already been mentioned above.

Arabic medicine had a profound influence on the emerging western world. Up to the 10th century the writings of ancient authors had for the most part fallen into oblivion in the West, and only in a few places were the early medieval Latin translations of some writings of Galen still in existence. The translations from Arabic into Latin of the old classical texts as well as of indigenous material during the 11th and 12th centuries laid the foundations of the "Arabism" in the medicine of the West. This trend was dominant for centuries, and was reversed only in modern times after long arguments. For long the rule held that he who would be a good physician must be a good Avicennist.

One must not judge the position of medicine in Islamic countries solely on the basis of the writings of the physicians. Physicians in any case were to be found only in the large cities, and most of the well known names were either personal doctors to the sultans or else professors. The urban poor and the rural population were practically deprived of all medical help.

The period from the 12th to the 17th centuries is chiefly one of decadence, contemporary with the decline of the caliphate, which was threatened internally by strife among the Arab dynasties and externally by the growing power of European cities.

A MOMENT
OF REFLECTION

There is no conclusion to this brief account of the epic evolution of the history of medicine. At the very moment where we halt, vast new vistas are opening up as medical science pushes the frontiers of knowledge forward. The most rapid advances in medicine have occurred within the life time of today's doctors.

In medicine as in science, the pure and the applied have progressed together over the years, the pure fertilising the applied with ideas, and the applied often providing the pure with the physical apparatus to help in the next intellectual leap forward. One may say that medical science is no more than the body of knowledge which is always being added on to by scientists, through controlled and reproducible observations. Medicine is a natural as well as social science, in the sense that it is concerned with human beings and is directed more immediately towards human welfare than any other natural science.

Modern science and medicine have immensely improved the lot of humanity. However, humanity can make use of these unimaginable powers for good or evil, but humanity has a major responsibility to insure that the world is safe for now and its future generations. Science and medicine are not standing still, and who can say how far the molecular biology, the chemistry or the physics of the future will have to adopt conceptions much more organicist than the atomic and mechanistic which have so far prevailed? Who knows what further developments of the psychosomatic conception in medicine's future advances may necessitate? In all such ways the thought complex of traditional Chinese sciences may yet have a much greater part to play in the future state of all sciences than might be admitted if science today was all that science will ever be.

Always we must remember that things are more complex than they seem, and that wisdom was not born with us, nor is it the property of any particular civilisation or people. The march of humanity in the study of Nature, of which humans are a part, is one single enterprise.

Further Reading

Bernal, J.D, *Science in History*, Penguin, Harmondsworth, 1969.

Brothwell, D and Sandison, A.T. (eds), *Diseases in Antiquity: A Survey of the Diseases, Injuries, and Surgery of Early Populations*, Charles Thomas, Springfield, 1967.

Huard, P and Wong, M, *Chinese Medicine*, Weidenfeld and Nicolson, London, 1968.

Koo, L.C, *Nourishment of Life: Health in Chinese Society*. Commercial Press, Hong Kong, 1982.

Nakayama, Yonezo, "La medicina en al antiguo Japon". In P. L. Entralgo, ed, *Historia universal de la medicina*, Vol. 1, Salvat Editores, Barcelona, 1975, pp. 205–225.

Nakayama, Shigeru-*Academic and Scientific Traditions in China, Japan and the West*, University of Tokyo Press, Tokyo, 1984.

Nakayama, Shigeru and Sivin, N (eds): *Chinese Science: Exploration of an Ancient Tradition*, MIT Press, Cambridge, Mass., 1973

Needham, J, *Science and Civilisation in China*, Cambridge University Press (1954, continuing) Approximately 30 volumes projected. The medical volume by Needham, J and Lu Gwei-Djen, with introductory notes by Sivin, N. is forthcoming.

Porkert, M, *The Theoretical Foundation of Chinese Medicine.*, MIT Press, Cambridge, Mass., 1974.

Temple, R.K.G, *China: Land of Discovery*, Stephens, Wellingborough, 1986.

Ullmann, M, *Islamic Medicine.*, University Press, Edinburgh, 1978.

Glossary of
Chinese Characters

Ajiatuo 阿伽陀
anbei 按背

Bencao gangmu 本草纲目
Bencao pinhui jingyao 本草品汇精要
Bencao shiyi 本草拾遗
Bencao tujing 本草图经
Bencao yanyi 本草衍义
Bencaojing jizhu 本草经集注
Bian, Que 扁鹊

Chan, Yuet Ling 陈月玲
Chao, Yuanfang 巢元方
Chen, Cangqi 陈藏器
chi 尺
Chiu, Ling Yeong 赵令扬
Chunyu, Yi 淳于意
cun 寸

Daguan bencao 大观本草
Dao 道
Dezong 德宗
di 地
dingshu 定数
dumai 督脉

Edo 江户
Eisai 荣西

fangshi 方士
Fuseya, Soteki 伏屋素狄
Fuying qianshuo 妇婴全说
fuzhen 腹诊

Ganjin 鉴真
ganmao 感冒
Ge, Hong 葛洪
geka 外科
Gengxin yuce 庚辛玉册
goseha 後世叶
guan 关
Guangjifang 广济方
Gujin lu yanfang 古今录验方
Gwee, Ah Leng 魏雅聆

Hanaoka, Seishû 华冈青洲
Hanlin yiguanyuan 翰林医官院
Heian 平安
Ho, P.Y. = Ho Peng Yoke 何丙郁
Hua, Shou 滑寿
Hua, Tuo 华陀
Huangfu, Mi 皇甫谧

Huangdi 黄帝
Huangdi neijing 黄帝内经
Huangdi neijing suwen 黄帝内经素问
Huihui yaofang 回回药方

Ishinô 医心方

Jianzhen 鉴真
Jiayou bencao 嘉祐本草
jing 经
Jinkui yaolue 金匮要略
Jiuhuang bencao 救荒本草

Kaibao bencao 开宝本草
Kaitai shinsho 解体新书
kexue 科学
Kim, Mu 金武
kinsôi 金疮医
Kissa yôjyôki 吃茶养身记
kohôha 古方叶
Kômô 红毛
Kou, Zongshi 寇宗奭

Lei, Xiao 雷敩
li (ceremony, propriety) 礼
li (pattern) 理
Li, Dongyuan 李东垣
Li, Gao 李杲
Li, Shizhen 李时珍
liangyi 兩仪
Lingshu 灵枢
lishu 历数
Liu, Wanshu 刘完素

Liu, Wentai 刘文泰
Longmeng 龙猛
Longshu 龙树
Lu, G.-D. = Lu Gwei-Djen 鲁桂珍
luo 络

mafeisan 麻沸散
mai 脉
Maijing 脉经
Majima 马岛
Mao, Zedong 毛泽东
Mawangdui 马王堆
Meiji 明治
Meng, Shen 孟洗
mingshu 命数
Mingyi bielu 明医别录
Miyashita, Saburô 宫下 三郎

Nakayama, Shigeru 中山 茂
Namban 南蛮
Naniwa 难波
Nara 奈良
Narabayashi, Chinzan 楢林 镇山
Neike xinshuo 内科新说
Ni, Weide 倪维德
Ningwan Zhu Quan jiqi Gengxin yuce 宁王朱权及其庚辛玉册

Peking Man = Beijing ren 北京人
Pujifang 普济方

qi 气
Qianjin fang 千金方
Qianjin yaofang 千金要方

Qianjin yifang 千金翼方
qie 切
qigong 气功
Qin, yueren 秦越人
Quanti xinbian 全体新编

ren (charity, benevolence, love, etc.) 仁
ren (human being) 人
renmai 任脉
Renzong 仁宗
ruyi 儒医
ryû 流

sancai 三才
Sanguo yanyi 三国演义
Sanron 产论
Sanshenggong 三圣宫
Seigan 清眼
Shanghan zabinglun 伤寒杂病论
Shanghanlun 伤寒论
Shen, Gua 沈括
Shennong 神农
Shennong bencaojing 神农本草经
shi 士
Shiji 史记
Shiliao bencao 食疗本草
Shisijing fahui 十四经发辉
Shôsôin 正仓院
Shôsôin yakubutsu 正仓院药物
shu 数
Sima, Qian 司马迁
Song, Ci 宋慈
Song, Jing 宋璟

Su, Dongpo 苏东坡
Su, Jing 苏敬
Su, Shi 苏轼
Su, Song 苏颂
Sugita, Gempaku 杉田 玄白
Sun Simiao 孙思邈
Suwen 素问

taichangbu 太常部
taiji 太极
taiyishu 太医署
Takeda, Syôkei 竹田 昌庆
Tamba, Yasuyori 丹波 康赖
Tang, Shenwei 唐慎微
Tao, Hongjing 陶弘景
Tashiro, Sanki 田代 三喜
tenyakuryo 典药寮
tian 天
tianshu 天数
Toba, Yu 拓跋郁
Tokugawa 德川
Tongren shuxuezhenjiu tujing 铜人腧穴针灸图经

wang 望
Wang, Andao 王安道
Wang, Bing 王冰
Wang, Chimin 王吉民
Wang, Haogu 王好古
Wang, Lü (also read Wang, Li) 王履
Wang, Shuhe 王叔和
Wang, Tao 王焘
Wang, Weiyi 王惟一
wen (auscultation and osphresis) 闻

wen (enquiring) 问
Wendi 文帝
wu 巫
Wu, Lien-teh 伍连德
wuxing 五行
wuyi 巫医

xianghua 相化
xiangke 相克
xiangsheng 相生
xiangzhi 相制
Xiao, Ziliang 萧子良
Xiaozong 孝宗
Xin, Gongyi 辛公义
Xinbian zhongyixue gaiyao 新编中医学概要
xing (form) 形
xing (element, phrase, agent) 行
Xinxiu bencao 新修本草
Xiuzhenfang 袖珍方
Xiyi luelun 西医略论
Xiyuanlu 洗冤录
Xuanzong 宣宗
xue 穴

Yang 阳
Yang, Jizhou 杨继洲
yanshe 验舌
Yaowang 药王
Yasuhiko, Asahina 朝比奈 泰彦
Yayoi 弥生
yi 义
yi zhe renshu 医者仁术
Yin 阴

yôka 痛科
Yu, Zhengxie 俞正燮
yunshu 运数

Zhang, Congzheng 张从正
Zhang, Ji 张机
Zhang, Qian 张骞
Zhang, Zhongjing 张仲景
Zhang, Zihe 张子和
Zhen Quan 甄权
Zhenglei bencao 证类本草
Zhenjiu daquan 针灸大全
Zhenjiu jiayijing 针灸甲乙经
Zhenyuan guanglifang 贞元广利方
zhi (wisdom, knowledge) 智
Zhichong 知聪
Zhongguo yixueshi jiangyi 中国医学史讲义
Zhouhou baiyifang 肘後百一方
Zhouhou jiuzufang 肘後救卒方
Zhoukoudian 周口店
Zhu, Quan 朱权
Zhu, Su 朱橚
Zhu, Xi 朱熹
Zhu, youdun 朱有燉
Zhuangzi 庄子
Zhubingyuan houlun 诸病源候论

Subject Index

Author Index